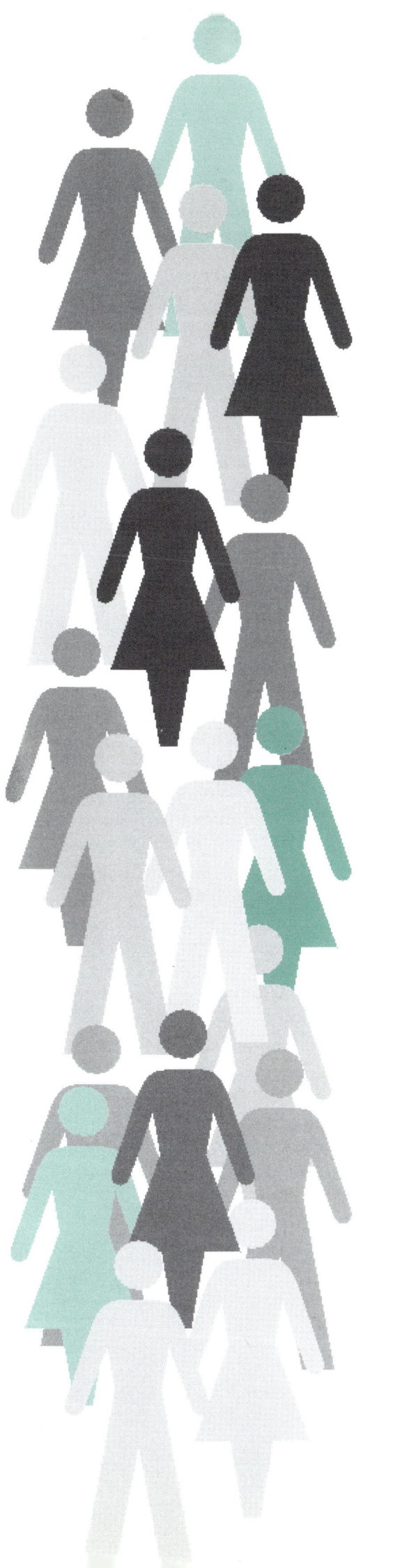

Don't Forget Us

Children with Learning Disabilities
and Severe Challenging Behaviour

Report of a Committee
set up by the Mental Health Foundation

© 1997 The Mental Health Foundation

ISBN 0 901944 42 4

The Mental Health Foundation
37 Mortimer Street
London W1N 7RJ

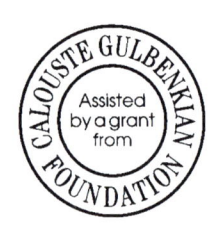

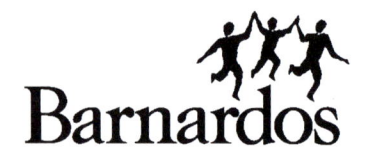

Assisted by a grant from Calouste Gulbenkian Foundation

Barnardos

The Mental Health Foundation wishes to thank the Calouste Gulbenkian Foundation and Barnardos for providing grants towards the production and dissemination of this report.

Design & print by Intertype

Membership of the Committee

Dr Philippa Russell OBE	Chair Director, The Council for Disabled Children and Associate Director, National Development Team for People with Learning Disabilities
Dr Jane Bernal	Senior Lecturer and Consultant Psychiatrist, St George's Hospital Medical School
Professor Eric Emerson	Professor of Clinical Psychology in Intellectual Disability, Hester Adrian Research Centre, University of Manchester
Matthew Griffiths	Inspector, The Further Education Funding Council
Dr John Harris	Chief Executive of the British Institute of Learning Disabilities
Christiana Horrocks	Formerly Social Services Inspector
Jean Jones	Education Advisor, MENCAP in Wales
Malcolm Jones	Chartered Psychologist and Headteacher at Progress School, part of Progress Education and Care Services. Formerly Chartered Psychologist at Beech Tree School
Dr Zarrina Kurtz	Consultant in Public Health and Health Policy. Formerly at South Thames Regional Health Authority
Michael Libby	Assistant Divisional Director, Barnados, London
Ron Ludgate	Strategic Director, Disability and Mental Health, London Borough of Brent
Professor Christine M Lyon	Professor of Common Law, Dean of the Faculty of Law and Director of the Centre for the Study of the Child, the Family and the Law, The University of Liverpool
Ruth Marchant	Development Manager, Charity Heritage
Peter Raine	Formerly Director, Social Services, London Borough of Brent
Peter Wilson	Director, Young Minds

Observers

Cedric Dowe	DfEE
Graham Holley	DfEE

Mental Health Foundation Staff Members

Tania Bronstein
Elizabeth Gale
Hazel Morgan
Cliff Prior

Editor

Alison Wertheimer

Contents

Membership of the Committee *opposite*
Foreword by Philippa Russell

1 Living with challenging behaviour

2 Introduction
2.1 Background *10*
2.2 Values and Principles *10*
2.3 Definitions *11*
2.4 How many children have learning disabilities and challenging behaviour? *13*
2.5 Why do some children with learning disabilities show severe challenging behaviour? *13*
References *16*
Appendix: some other relevant definitions *17*

3 Developing community-based services and family support
3.1 The challenge of inclusion *18*
3.2 The whole family *19*
3.3 Family support *20*
3.4 Informal support *21*
3.5 Teamwork *21*
3.6 Parents as team members *22*
3.7 Short-term care *23*
3.8 Emergency care *24*
Recommendations *24*
References *25*

4 The rôle of education services
4.1 Background *26*
4.2 Definitions *27*
4.3 Early intervention *27*
4.4 A 'whole school' approach *27*
4.5 Responding to children with severe learning disabilities who present challenging behaviour *28*
4.6 Children with emotional and behavioural difficulties *30*
4.7 Exclusion of pupils with challenging behaviour *30*
4.8 Residential education *31*
4.9 Parent participation *32*
Recommendations *32*
References *33*

5 Away from home: residential provision
5.1 Introduction *35*
5.2 Criteria for use of residential provision *35*
5.3 Current use of residential provision *36*
5.4 Residential provision and collaboration *36*
5.5 Secure accommodation *37*
5.6 The legal basis for use of secure accommodation *37*
5.7 The impact of privatisation *38*
Recommendation *38*
References *39*

6 Treatments
6.1 Introduction *40*
6.2 Timing of treatment *42*
6.3 Multi-disciplinary, multi-agency assessment *43*
6.4 Where is treatment provided? *44*
6.5 Families *44*
6.6 Choice of treatment(s) *45*
6.7 Treatment approaches *47*
6.8 Alternative or complementary treatments *52*
Recommendations *52*
References *53*

Contents continued overleaf

7   The legal framework and other legal issues

   The legal framework for support services *55*
7.1   Introduction *55*
7.2   Part III Children Act (1989) and Part I Schedule 2 *55*
7.3   Legislative provision in Scotland and Northern Ireland *59*
   Other legal issues *60*
7.4   Background to issues of care, control and safety *60*
7.5   Challenges and dilemmas *60*
7.6   The current legal framework for care, control and safety *61*
7.7   Basic principles governing the care of children *62*
7.8   Parental responsibility: provision of care, control and safety *62*
7.9   Control and restraint *63*
7.10   Relevant government departmental guidance *65*
7.11   Medical treatment *66*
7.12   Key principles *66*
   Recommendations *66*
   References *67*

8   Commissioning and purchasing in the health service: assessment and planning in social services

   Commissioning and purchasing in the health service *68*
8.1   Principles *68*
8.2   The current situation *68*
8.3   Challenges for specialist services *69*
8.4   Guidance on commissioning and purchasing of specialist services *69*
8.5   Commissioning and purchasing rôles *70*
8.6   Developing an informed approach *71*
8.7   Issues in contracting *72*
8.8   From extra-contractual referrals – to a strategic approach *72*
8.9   Collaborative commissioning *73*
   Assessment and planning in social services *74*
8.10   A common framework *74*
8.11   A changing environment in children's services: purchaser/provider issues in planning *74*
8.12   Mapping needs and resources *75*
8.13   Assessment issues *76*
8.14   Building consumers into the planning framework *79*
   Recommendations *80*
   References *81*

Epilogue *82*

Overarching recommendations *85*

Appendix 1
The conduct and activities of the Committee *86*

Appendix 2
Individuals and organisations submitting evidence *87*

Foreword

by Philippa Russell

This report has been produced in response to the Mental Health Foundation's growing concern about the situation of children with learning disabilities and severe challenging behaviour. During the last few years, the Foundation has become increasingly aware of significant shortcomings in services to these children and their families.

With the recent debates about the much larger numbers of non-disabled children with emotional and behavioural difficulties and widespread media coverage of issues such as juvenile crime and school exclusions, there was a grave danger that the needs of this highly vulnerable group of children and young people would be overlooked.

The Committee was established in October 1993 with the following terms of reference:

'To review and report on services for children with learning disabilities and severe challenging behaviour; and make recommendations for the future development of services.'

The Mental Health Foundation was particularly concerned that children with learning disabilities and severe challenging behaviour should be seen as 'children first'. They and their families should be accorded both respect and access to good quality child-focused services. During the course of its work, the Committee was in no doubt that unless children with learning disabilities and severe challenging behaviour receive appropriate support and services, they experience a real risk of exclusion not only from children's services such as schools, playgroups or play and leisure activities, but from the experience of family life itself.

However, despite the considerable concerns expressed to the Committee about the impact on families and services of severe challenging behaviour, we received important messages about the children themselves. Parents and professionals emphasised the value they placed on the children concerned and emphasised their essential humanity. As one parent commented:

'My child challenges us all as a family. Sometimes we feel under tremendous strain. But John is still our child. He gives us pleasure, we have things we can enjoy together, we believe we have a future. What we treasure are those professionals, those friends and family members who are willing to work with us. They see our son as a special family member not a nuisance who is too 'expensive' or 'difficult'. Don't forget that children with learning disabilities and severely challenging behaviour are children and don't try and exclude them from community and society.'

However, if children like John are to remain with their families and local communities and enjoy the positive experiences of education, play and socialisation available to their peers, they require a comprehensive and coordinated range of support services including, in some instances, very specialist interventions.

The Foundation's decision to set up the Committee was given added impetus by the publication of the Department of Health's review of services for adults with learning disabilities and challenging behaviour (the Mansell Report, 1993) which expressed the view that *'much severe challenging behaviour starts in childhood'* (Mansell, 1993). This strengthened the Foundation's belief that the needs of these children must be examined as a priority.

The Committee's task has been difficult at times, reflecting in no small measure the complexities of the issues. One of the most striking features of our work has been the enormous complexity of the service system involved, the many different agencies who have a part to play and the range of professionals and types of services which are needed.

The children's problems are often complex too. Although numerically they are not a large group, they present a range of different and often 'low incidence' disabilities. Our understanding of the causes and origins of challenging behaviour in childhood is limited and opinions are often divided as to how best to assess the needs and decide on the most appropriate interventions.

At the same time, we have been aware of the opportunities offered by some of the major changes which have taken place in children's services over the past decade. The legal framework enshrined in the Children Act (1989) and the spirit of entitlement to a broad and balanced education reflected in the Education Act (1996) offer new possibilities to children with learning disabilities and severe challenging behaviour.

The Committee has therefore sought both to highlight shortcomings in current services for these children and also to suggest positive ways of moving forward, building on the opportunities offered by recent changes in legislation, policy and practice.

Our work as a Committee would not have been possible without the invaluable support and guidance of many individuals and organisations. In particular we would like to thank the Foundation's staff: Elizabeth Gale, Tania Bronstein, Hazel Morgan, Cliff Prior and Suzanne Kenny for their unlimited commitment, patience and practical help throughout the Committee's working life. The contributions of Alison Wertheimer and Val Bull, Adminstrator at the Council for Disabled Children, have been invaluable.

We greatly appreciated those who commented on or gave advice or evidence to the Committee. We are indebted to the families who shared their experience of learning disability and severe challenging behaviour for their honesty and courage in telling us about their lives. To ensure their confidentiality, we have changed names and some personal details, when drawing upon their stories throughout the text. Professor Peter Hill, Dr Ian McKinlay, Tom McLean, Professor Jim Mansell, Rowena Rossiter and David Tobin read and made many useful comments on the draft report.

As Chair of the Committee, I must express our real gratitude for the commitment, time and energy which the individual members of the Committee brought to our work. All the Committee members had busy professional lives and many other pressures on their time. But their enthusiasm and vision of how services could be developed for this particularly challenging group of children were remarkable. It was a privilege for me as Chair to work with them.

CHAPTER 1
Living with challenging behaviour

Much of this report focuses on the services, treatments and interventions which are needed in order to support and assist children with learning disabilities and severe challenging behaviour and their families. Inevitably organisational structures and processes dominate the discussion at times, but we must never lose sight of these children and their families and the reality of 'living with challenging behaviour'. Indeed, some of the most compelling evidence we received was from parents, describing their day-to-day lives.

The Committee makes no apology for starting this report with some snapshots of the lives of these children, of their brothers and sisters and parents. What is it like to live with 'challenging behaviour' twenty-four hours a day – whether it is your own or that of another member of your family?

The Committee is also hoping to show something of what lies behind the term 'challenging behaviour' - a description which emphasises that some people (including children) behave in ways which present a significant challenge to services. The motivation behind this change in terminology was laudable: services have too often laid the blame for their failures at the door of those they purported to serve, rather than acknowledging their own shortcomings and their inability to 'meet the challenge'.

The intention was also to present a more positive image: people were no longer to be described as having 'problems' or 'difficulties'. Yet the day-to-day lives of many children with challenging behaviour – and their families – are difficult, are full of problems. Indeed, many families would describe their situation in much stronger language.

The children and young people who are the subject of this report are seen as presenting challenges to others, but we cannot minimise the distress and misery experienced by children like Mary, David and James.

'Mary beats her head with her fists; she has already blinded herself in the left eye and the right one is developing cataracts.'

'Daniel is held down or tied up most of the time.'

'James has been very badly treated in the past. One particular form of 'therapy' appears to have made him terrified of most adults. He strips his clothes off, cowers in the corner of his bedroom and screams that the door should be locked. If people he does not trust try to enter his room he furiously beats his head on the floor and walls. He bleeds extensively and becomes excessively distressed.'

The behaviour of one child can also cause enormous distress to other children in the family. Parents faced with competing demands often have to resort to restraint in order to make life more bearable for the family as a whole, but are uncomfortably aware of making unacceptable compromises.

'Penny is our fourth child ... [She is] so active and so dangerous. She'll climb anything and she screams all the time. My other children can't stand it. When the holidays come and they are in and out, I lock her in her room. I don't leave her long. But if I have something to do I lock her up. The school was horrified when I told them. I said: 'Come and see my flat. If she fell and killed herself, you'd be after me then.'

Any parent can find it upsetting if their child is isolated and has no friends. Thankfully for most children this is often a temporary phase, perhaps when starting at a new school or moving to a new neighbourhood. For Donald and his mother isolation has become a way of life, but the rejection and loneliness are nonetheless extremely painful:

'My son ... used to go to a holiday play scheme but that has all stopped. There were other children with learning disabilities who were quite frail. The staff thought Donald might trample over them.

You don't know what it's like to have a child nobody wants. When Donald goes to school I always try to make myself invisible in the playground. I feel the other parents will be pointing fingers at me all the time – there's the mother of the child nobody wants. It's just me and Donald and it's very lonely.'

Going out, into what one parent describes as 'the real world', can be difficult. Even just going to the shops can be a fraught experience for families like Stephen's and Judy's:

'Because Stephen grew so big and ran so fast we stopped taking him out.'

'It's when I take Judy out [that] it all goes wrong. She's fine until something upsets her. Then she scratches and bites ... and she nearly bit an old man the other day. He had a black hat and she doesn't like black hats.'

If taking a child out is too difficult, families may be forced to spend more time at home. But trying to create a comfortable pleasant home can be hard, as Sammy's mother discovered:

'I think he's in the wheelchair too much. He can walk, but he wrecks everything. I know it's selfish but I don't want to live in a house where everything is wrecked.'

Although so-called 'normal' family life may be hard to define, when one child has challenging behaviour, families can end up with a highly 'abnormal' existence. Everyone's lifestyle may be dictated by the needs of the child with behavioural difficulties. But even when help is made available, it may impose demands on the family which make an ordinary life virtually impossible. Some kind of structured intervention may be the only way that the family can continue to function, but at what cost?

'Our lives are utterly abnormal because of the pressures of compliance with different professionals' expectations. Sometimes I feel we live in a programme not a home. If you were a child, would you want to come home to a programme? I have no time for John's siblings. And he has no time to be a child.'

The Committee heard from many parents about being on the receiving end of multiple sources of advice. Some families had seen as many as twenty professionals in one year. As one parent commented:

'You try partnership ... it's like Noah's ark.'

Some families felt they had been subject to 'onslaughts' of treatment with no one explaining the rationale for them or the possible outcomes.

'I don't want to be a cheap treatment resource, always there at any time of day or night. It wouldn't matter if they didn't all give me programmes for my child. Aggregated they institutionalise our days as a family. We don't feel ourselves to be in that horrid phase 'a handicapped family', except that our lives are utterly abnormal because of the pressure of compliance with different professionals' expectations.'

In some cases there was a real risk of expert advice and support being negated because of a lack of collaboration in planning and intervention. As one parent suggested:

'Couldn't professionals work as a team to help all of us prioritise what services we are going to use and which treatment we will all try?'

The Committee's impression was that an increasing number of parents are saying that they want to be 'parents first' – or at the very least to be able to negotiate their rôle in treatment programmes. They want a relationship with professionals in which they feel valued and respected. They want to be able to negotiate how, when and where they will participate in programmes with their child. They want to be given explanations and not instructions:

'Sometimes we may have a particular priority for a behaviour which is not yours: ask us. Enabling a child to travel on the bus or to give parents some sleep may be the key to a lot more participation and a much more supportive family. Equally all of us feel strongly about prioritising interventions for behaviours which might exclude our children from school.'

Parents and professionals may have very different lifestyles. Some parents felt that treatment interventions were being proposed which were based on the assumption that families had carpeting and soundproofing, separate bedrooms, a car and a telephone, one parent at home all day and no siblings with competing demands:

'I wish the professionals would really think about how we balance quality, safety, personal preferences within very different family lifestyles and expectations. You feel you always have to fit the services if you have a child with challenging behaviour.'

In many cases a number of different interventions will need to be tried out, evaluated, pursued or rejected. Severe challenging behaviour may persist over time and all treatments and interventions will require constant evaluation and, if necessary, revision. Parents can feel very demoralised by having to persist with treatment which does not appear to be working. They feel inadequate, as though they are failing not only their child but the professionals too. Disappointments are inevitable; knowledge about the best ways of treating children with challenging behaviour is often incomplete. But parents could cope better if there was a supportive relationship. One parent commented:

'Tell us if the treatment may not work ... be sad with us if it doesn't, but show commitment to trying again. Keep us in the picture about how and why you want us to work.'

Another parent reminded us that:

'Children with learning disabilities and severely challenging behaviour may be seen as 'too complicated' and 'too expensive' by conventional children's services. But we love our children and see them as worthy of the best possible support. Also, if we have to talk 'value for money', let's remember that there are social and economic costs to failing to make proper provision for challenging behaviour.'

CHAPTER 2 Introduction

2.1 Background

The Committee began its work with strong messages from the Department of Health's review of services for adults with learning disabilities and challenging behaviour or mental health problems (1993). The Mansell Report raised important concerns about the commissioning, purchasing and provision of services for adults with learning disabilities and challenging behaviour and clearly stated the importance of looking at children's services in order to understand the antecedents of any challenging behaviour and to improve the quality and coherence of provision. Early evidence to the Committee identified four key issues, which were frequently pressure points for families, professionals and commissioners. These were substantiated in evidence subsequently received and provided a key agenda for the Committee's subsequent work.

These key issues (all of which merit priority action) were:

- Major concerns about the current fragmentation, duplication and poor coordination of assessment and support services offered to many families. Aspirations to integrate assessment arrangements and develop joint case management and commissioning arrangements were frequently unmet. Several reports on 'children in need' (in particular the Audit Commission's report Seen but not Heard (1993)) had highlighted the challenge of balancing services designed to promote the 'well-being' of all children, with the special and additional needs of children with more complex disabilities or medical conditions.

- The need for development of central government policy about children in general to pay more attention to meeting the requirements of children with the most complex needs, in inclusive settings wherever possible. It should also assist the full range of local services to identify their complementary contributions within widespread debate both about how best to develop local policy and practice within a coherent strategic framework and about the balance of inclusive and specialist services for children with the most complex needs.

- The need to develop a coherent and strategic approach to planning local services, which ensures that children with learning disabilities and severe challenging behaviour receive well coordinated services, with commissioning arrangements reflecting both good quality child care practice and access to specialist services as appropriate.

- The importance of training for all staff working with children with learning disabilities and challenging behaviour, to ensure a strategic approach and inter-agency agreement on curriculum and core competencies.

2.2 Values and principles

We were clear from the start that the work of the Committee should be based on a set of clearly articulated principles and values, that suggest goals towards which services should strive. In particular, our work has been informed throughout by the values underlying the UN Convention on the Rights of the Child (1989), to which the British government is a signatory.

The UN Convention explicitly recognises that children are a vulnerable group who are entitled to special care and assistance. The Convention sets out important principles, namely:

- the need for any decision to be based on the best interests of the child;
- respect for the child's privacy and dignity;
- the need to listen to children's views;
- enabling children to enjoy the highest attainable standards of health and development;
- the right to education;
- the right to treatment;

- special care for disabled children;
- protection against negligence and cruelty;
- the right, as far as possible, to a family life.

The Convention applies to all children 'without discrimination', but Article 23 specifically addresses the rights of the disabled child:

'… to enjoy a full and decent life, in conditions which ensure dignity, promote self-reliance and facilitate the child's active participation in the community.'

It also states

'the right of the disabled child to special care, education, health care; … all these shall be designed in a manner conducive to the child achieving the fullest possible social integration and individual development.'

The Committee firmly supports the rights of children with learning disabilities and challenging behaviour as set out in Article 23.

The values and principles expressed in the UN Convention on the Rights of the Child are fully consistent with 'Ordinary Life' values (Blunden & Allen, 1987; King's Fund, 1980, 1984, 1989) and the notion of 'service accomplishments' (O'Brien 1987) which have had a powerful influence in services for adults with learning disabilities over the last decade.

'Ordinary life' principles would argue that every child with learning disabilities:

- has the same human value as anyone else in the community;
- has a right and a need to live like other children as part of their local community;
- is an individual.

John O'Brien (1987) has suggested that these underlying values can be translated into five 'accomplishments' to which services should aim:

- Community Presence: which would include the opportunity to use the services, be in the same places and share the experiences which constitute community life for most children and families.
- Choice: through extending the range of choices available to children and their families.
- Competence: by supporting people in learning and using meaningful and useful new skills relevant to their daily life.
- Respect: valuing people and respecting them as individuals in their own right.
- Relationships: enabling people to form and sustain positive and stable relationships.

2.3 Definitions

Many different (and sometimes overlapping) terms are used to describe the children who are the subject of this report. Different professional groups and agencies have their own terms and definitions. Acts of Parliament and their associated guidelines and circulars also employ a range of terms, usually reflecting the terminology preferred by whichever government department sponsored the legislation.

The children who are the subject of this report may be described at different times and by different services or professionals as having:

- challenging behaviours;
- learning disabilities;
- learning difficulties;
- special educational needs;
- mental health problems;
- [and be children] in need.

We will focus here on 'challenging behaviour' and 'learning disability' since this is most directly relevant to our work. But we recognise that these children will also be defined as having 'learning difficulties' and thus 'special educational needs' and will also be children 'in need', under the Children Act (1989).

2.3.1 Learning disability

The term 'learning disability' has generally replaced the term 'mental handicap'. It is most commonly used within health and social services. The DoH defines 'learning disability' as a:

▶ reduced ability to understand new or complex information, to learn new skills (impaired intelligence); and

▶ reduced ability to cope independently (impaired social functioning);

▶ which started before adulthood with a lasting effect on development' (DoH 1995).

The term 'learning disability', as we are using it, also refers to children who in education would often be described as having a 'learning difficulty'. The Education Act (1993) and Code of Practice (1993) define the child with learning difficulties as one who:

▶ has significantly greater difficulty in learning than the majority of children of the same age;

▶ has a disability which either prevents or hinders the child from making use of educational facilities of a kind provided for children of the same age in schools within the LEA;

▶ is under five and falls within the above definitions or would do so if special educational provision was not made for the child.

It needs to be kept in mind that the term 'learning disability' will include children with very different types and degrees of disabilities. Some children with learning disabilities will only need a moderate amount of support to make the best of the opportunities open to them in ordinary schools. Other children will have profound and multiple disabilities. They may, in addition to their severe learning disabilities, also have physical or sensory impairments or epilepsy.

2.3.2 Severe Challenging behaviour

The term challenging behaviour has generally replaced the terms 'problem behaviour' or 'disturbed behaviour'. It is now commonly used within education, health and social services. ·

The Committee based its work on the most commonly adopted definition (Emerson et al, 1987, 1988):

'Severely challenging behaviour refers to behaviour of such an intensity, frequency or duration that the physical safety of the person or others is likely to be placed in serious jeopardy, or behaviour which is likely to seriously limit or deny access to and use of ordinary community facilities.'

But the Committee also recognised that there were issues more specifically relating to children, so we expanded the definition to include the following:

[or] 'behaviour which is likely to impair a child's personal growth, development and family life and which represents a challenge to services, to families and to the children themselves, however caused.'

The term 'challenging behaviour' generally refers to behaviours which have a negative impact on the child's social or physical surroundings. These behaviours will range from socially disruptive behaviours, such as persistent screaming, aggressive and destructive behaviours, to behaviours such as self-injury (eg hitting the head against a hard surface or poking the eyes) which can endanger the physical and/or emotional well-being of the child or young person.

Any attempt to define 'challenging' or 'problem' behaviour needs to acknowledge that judgements about what is challenging or problematic will be based on wide variety of different perspectives and experiences. What is the likely impact of acting in a potentially 'challenging' way for that specific child, their family, their school, other service providers and their particular community? For schools, what may be regarded as challenging by one teacher may not challenge another. Similarly families will have different perceptions of what kinds of behaviour are more or less acceptable or challenging. Certainly, a family who pride themselves on keeping their home tidy and immaculate will be likely to find a child who damages furniture and fittings more challenging than a family where material possessions are seen as less important.

Severe challenging behaviours are, however, likely to result in adverse consequences for a wide range of people:

▶ **For the child**, some challenging behaviours, such as self-injuring, can threaten their health or even their life. Behaviours, such as aggression, can rapidly lead to the child's rejection and exclusion. Other behaviours, such as stereotypy or overactivity may, over time, restrict personal growth and seriously impair the development of personal relationships.

▶ **For the child's family**, caring for a son or daughter with severe challenging behaviour is likely to have a profound effect upon their day-to-day life. Families often talk of the emotional and physical exhaustion resulting from bringing up a child with severe challenging behaviour. They may become cut off from friendships and activities in the wider community. For a significant number of families, the demands of caring can lead to them feeling there is no alternative, but to request a residential placement for their son or daughter.

▶ **For education, health and social services**, children who pose a danger to themselves, or others, often challenge schools and other services. Supporting such children often places considerable demands on skills, time and resources. All too often, the response to such demands is to exclude the child and to seek a placement in a specialised residential school. This may be particularly likely when professionals are unsure of the legality of particular controls or treatments.

▶ **For the wider community**, socially unacceptable behaviours are likely to elicit avoidance by and exclusion from the community.

2.4 How many children have learning disabilities and challenging behaviour?

There are no hard and fast figures which allow us to estimate either how many children have a learning disability, or how many of these show challenging behaviour.

Very crudely, it is likely that approximately two and a half per cent of the population have some degree of learning disability (Zigler and Hodap, 1986) and that 0.6 per cent of children will have a severe learning disability (Kavanagh & Opit, 1996). The British Paediatric Association (1994) estimates that, in an 'average' area with a population of 250,000 people, there will be:

▶ 200 children with severe learning disabilities and that;

▶ 15-20 children with severe learning disabilities will be born each year.

There is very little agreement about how many children with learning disabilities are likely to show challenging behaviour. As we have already indicated, the term 'challenging behaviour' is open to a number of interpretations and what may be challenging in one setting may not be challenging in another.

Studies undertaken in the UK illustrate the range and diversity of 'challenging' behaviours which can occur amongst children and young people with learning disabilities:

▶ Chris and Diana Kiernan (1994) looked at challenging behaviour in 68 schools for children with severe learning difficulties. Just over 8 per cent of pupils were identified as 'extremely' difficult or 'very difficult' to manage and a further 14 per cent presented challenges of a lesser nature. Projected to a national level, these figures suggest that around 2,000 pupils in England and Wales present a serious challenge and a further 3,400 a lesser challenge.

▶ Chris Kiernan and colleagues (eg Kiernan & Qureshi, 1993) have been involved in a series of studies looking at the nature of challenging behaviours. The results from these studies suggest that, in an 'average' area with a population of 250,000 people, there will be approximately 25 children with learning disabilities who show at least one form of challenging behaviour which poses a 'serious' management problem or would do, if it were not for specific measures undertaken to control the behaviour (eg locked doors, reinforced windows, avoiding particular activities). Of these, 12 children would be considered to show 'more severe' challenging behaviour. The table and figures on page 14 illustrate some aspects of the situation and characteristics of these children.

2.5 Why do some children with learning disabilities show severe challenging behaviour?

As we have seen, the term 'challenging behaviour' covers a wide range of specific behaviours. Some of these (eg temper tantrums) are also common among children who do not have learning disabilities. Others, for example repetitive severe self-injury, are very unusual among their non-learning disabled peers. Not surprisingly, given the range of behaviours covered by the term, there is no one 'cause' of challenging behaviour.

The Committee is aware that the origins of challenging behaviour are likely to be

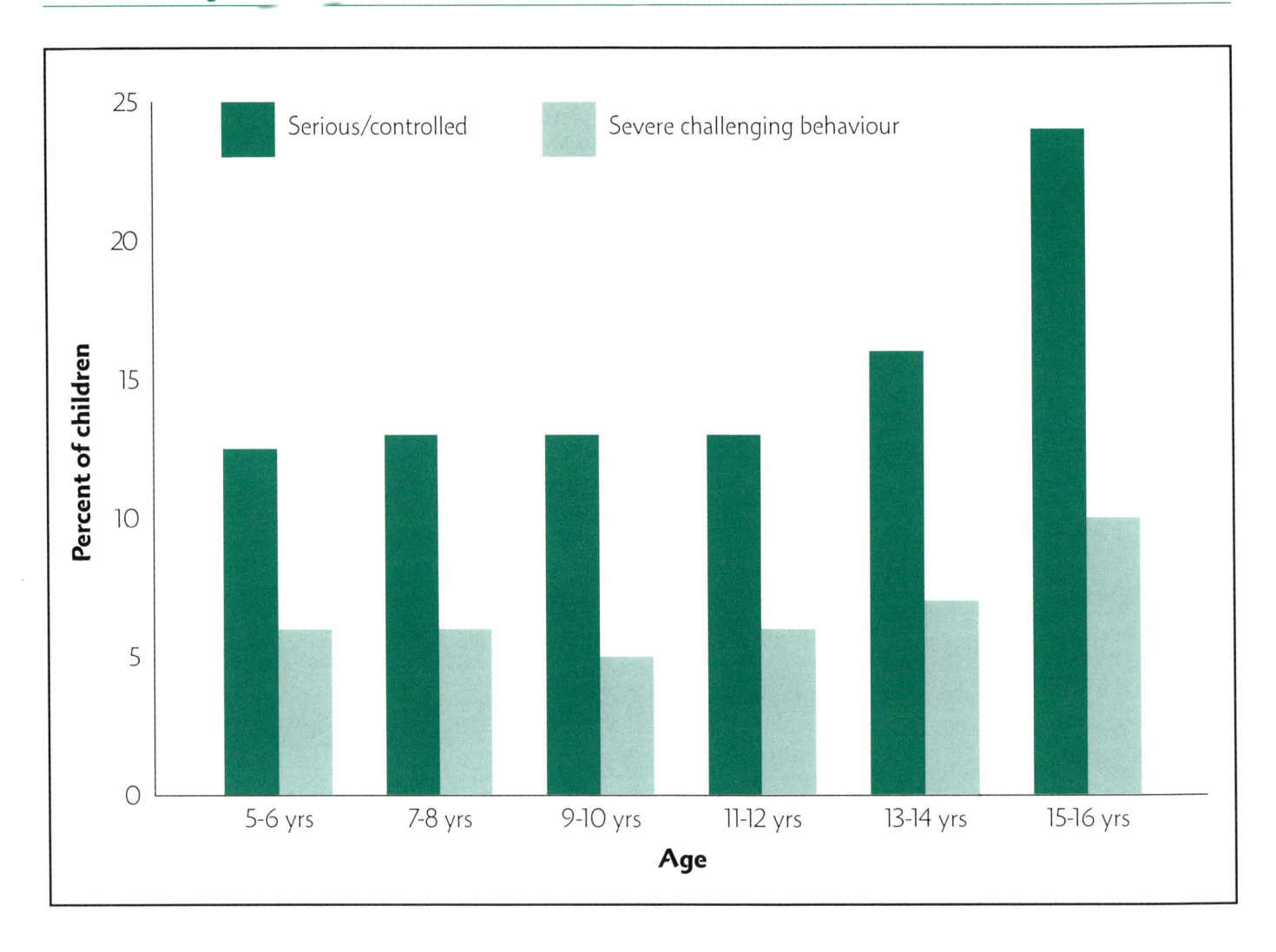

Some Aspects of the Situation and Characteristics of Children Who Show Challenging Behaviour

	Percent of all children with challenging behaviour	Percent of children with severe challenging behaviour
boys	69%	70%
have epilepsy	33%	37%
have visual impairment	26%	24%
have hearing impairment	17%	17%
have visual and hearing impairment	10%	9%
incontinent	55%	35%
need help with eating	42%	31%
need help with dressing	66%	61%
show 'serious or controlled' aggression	51%	68%
show 'serious or controlled' self-injury	33%	37%
show 'serious or controlled' destructive behaviours	38%	56%
show 'serious or controlled' other forms of challenging behaviour	80%	82%
show 'serious or controlled' challenging behaviors in two or more of the above four areas	37%	52%

complex and in many cases will not have a single cause. We also appreciate that we still have much to learn about the causes of challenging behaviour and are aware that the contents of this section are likely to present an incomplete picture. We feel that it is important, however, that we continue building on existing knowledge in order to develop more appropriate and effective ways of supporting children who 'challenge' themselves, their families, their schools and the wider community.

It is possible to draw a number of very general conclusions from existing knowledge. We have tried to summarise some of the more important of these below:

▶ **Challenging behaviours often emerge in early childhood**, but may not become 'severe' until the child becomes older when increasing physical size can make management more difficult and behaviours which may be broadly acceptable in very young children (stripping or having tantrums, for example,) becomes less socially acceptable, particularly outside the family home.

▶ **Some children are more 'at risk' of developing challenging behaviours than others.** For example, boys are more likely than girls to show 'outer-directed' challenging behaviours such as aggression. Children with physical and/or sensory impairments and children with autism and other specific syndromes are more likely to show challenging behaviour.

> Autism is a permanent condition which arises during infancy or childhood and is characterised by impaired social interaction, delayed or deviant language development and a preference for sameness, as shown by stereotyped play patterns, abnormal preoccupations or resistance to change. Autism often occurs in association with learning disability, but it can also be present without any additional intellectual impairment. (Harris J, Allen D et al, 1996) (see also page 17)

▶ **Some environments or experiences may be more 'at risk' of leading to the development or exacerbation of challenging behaviour than others.** For example, children with learning disabilities may, like their non-disabled peers, be more likely to develop challenging behaviour following inadequate or inappropriate early parenting, premature separation, abuse or material and social deprivation.

▶ **Much challenging behaviour serves an important function for the child.** In many cases, challenging behaviours are one of the ways in which the child exerts their influence or control over their world. For example, challenging behaviour may be one of the ways in which a child elicits the attention of carers or escapes from tasks or activities they find distressing. In this sense, much challenging behaviour is 'communicative' and, at least in the short-term, 'adaptive'. In other instances, challenging behaviours may be rewarding to the child because of their 'internal' consequences. Many examples of stereotyped behaviours seem to be ways in which the child with severe learning disabilities can provide some stimulation for themselves when bored. Some forms of self-injury may trigger the release of morphine-like substances in the brain.

▶ **Undiagnosed and untreated medical conditions may indirectly lead to challenging behaviour.** For example, the resulting pain and discomfort from ear infections may find expression in repeated challenging behaviour (eg screaming or head-banging), at least in part because discomfort and pain are likely to increase the importance to them of interactions with carers.

▶ **Some examples of challenging behaviour may be related to an underlying psychiatric or neurological disorder.** It is clear that not all challenging behaviour is purely 'functional'. Some examples of challenging behaviour may be related to epilepsy or neurobiological changes associated with particular syndromes. Others may be a reflection of an underlying psychiatric disorder.

This is obviously an incomplete and necessarily superficial look at the causes or origins of challenging behaviour. It does, however, illustrate an extremely important issue – that challenging behaviour is a particularly complex phenomenon to which there are unlikely to be any simple or easy answers. Only by working together in a true partnership between families, professionals, managers and policy makers are we likely to make significant headway. It is to this task that we now turn.

References

Blunden R and Allen D (1987). Facing the Challenge: An Ordinary Life for People with Learning Difficulties and Challenging Behaviours. King's Fund, London.

British Paediatric Association (1994). Services for Children and Adolescents with Learning Disability (Mental Handicap). Report of a British Paediatric Association Working Party.

Department of Health (1995). The Health of the Nation: A Strategy for People with Learning Disabilities. London, DoH.

Emerson E, Toogood A, Massell J, Barrett S, Bell C, Cummings R and McCool C (1987). 'Challenging behaviour and community services: 1 introduction and overview'. Mental Handicap 15:166-9.

Emerson E, Cummings R, Barrett S, Hughes H, McCool C and Toogood A (1988). 'Challenging behaviour and community services 2: who are the people who challenge services?' Mental Handicap 16:16-19.

Harris J, Allen D, Cornick M, Jefferson A and Mills R (1996). Physical Interventions: A Policy Framework. British Institute of Learning Disabilities. National Autistic Society.

Kavanagh S and Opit E (1996) The Prevalence Balance of Care Costs and Cost-Effectiveness of Care for People with Learning Disabilities in Great Britain. Personal Social Services Research Unit, University of Kent.

Kiernan C and Kiernan D (1994) 'Challenging behaviour in schools for pupils with severe learning difficulties'. Mental Handicap Research 7:117-201.

Kiernan C and Qureshi H (1993) 'Challenging behaviour' in: Research to Practice? Implications of Research on the Challenging Behaviour of People with Learning Disabilities Ed. C Kiernan. British Institute of Learning Disabilities.

King's Fund (1980). An Ordinary Life: Comprehensive Locally-Based Residential Services for Mentally Handicapped People. King's Fund Centre, London.

King's Fund (1984). An Ordinary Life and Treatment under Security for People with Mental Handicap. King's Fund Centre, London.

O'Brien J (1987). 'A guide to life style planning using the activities catalogue to integrate services and natural support systems' in: The Activity Catalogue: An Alternative Curriculum for Youth and Adults with Severe Disabilities Ed. B W Wilcox & G T Bellamy. Brookes, Baltimore.

Zigler E and Hodap R M (1986). Understanding Mental Retardation. Cambridge University Press, Cambridge.

Appendix to Chapter 2
Some other relevant definitions

Special educational needs (Part III, Education Act (1993), now Education Act 1996)

A child has special educational needs if he or she has a learning difficulty as defined above which calls for special educational provision to be made.

Children in need (Children Act (1989))

All children with learning disabilities and challenging behaviour will be children in need. A child in need is defined as one:

- who is unlikely, or does not have the opportunity, to achieve or maintain a reasonable standard of health or development without provision made by the local authority;
- whose health and development are likely to be significantly impaired or further impaired without the provision of services by the local authority;
- is disabled.

Emotional and behavioural difficulties (DFEE Circulars on Pupils with Problems, Circular No. 2 December 1993)

The term 'emotional and behavioural difficulties' is sometimes used interchangeably, but inaccurately, with 'challenging behaviour'.

'Emotional and behavioural difficulties range from social maladaptation to abnormal emotional stresses. They are persistent ... and constitute learning difficulties ... . They may become apparent through withdrawn, passive, depressive, aggressive or self-injurious tendencies. They may have a single or a number of causes and may be associated with school, family or other environments or physical or sensory impairments ... emotional and behavioural difficulties are caused by many interacting factors ... . Rates are likely to be greater ... [among] children with other learning, health or developmental difficulties.'

Autism – an additional definition

Autism and related disorders are relatively common among children with learning disabilities.

Autism can be defined as a developmental disorder, first manifest under the age of three in which there is:

- Qualitative impairment in reciprocal social interaction;
- Qualitative impairment in verbal and non-verbal communication and in imaginative activity;
- Marked restricted repertoire of activities and interests.

This definition, which is based on that in ICD 10 and DSM IV has wide international support. There is a larger group of children, who meet some but not all the criteria of autistic disorder. These children are variously referred to as showing 'pervasive developmental disorder' (DSM IV) and 'atypical autism' (ICD10), 'autistic features' 'on the autistic spectrum' 'wider autistic phenotype' or 'Wing's triad'. The triad, which consists of social impairments associated with abnormalities in the use of speech and very restricted interests, may occur in more than half of all children with severe learning disabilities.

Children with autism and related disorders often develop challenging behaviour, which may be persistent and disabling. Many of the children the committee visited at two highly specialised schools for children with learning disabilities and severely challenging behaviour also met criteria for autism.

Services for children with learning disabilities and severely challenging behaviour must be aware of the particular needs of children with autism. (Dr Jane Bernal)

Wing L and Gould J (1979) Severe impairments of social interaction and associated abnormalities in children epidemiology and classification. Journal of Autism and Development Disorders, 9: 11-30.

Rutter M Bailey A J Bolton P and Le Couteur (1994) Autism and known medical conditions: myth and substance. Journal of Child Psychology and Psychiatry 35: 311-322.

World Health Organisation (1992) the ICD-10 Classification of Mental and Behavioural Disorders Research Criteria. Geneva, World Health Organisation.

Wing L (1993) The definition and prevalence of autism. A review. European Child & Adolescent Psychiatry 2: 61-74.

American Psychiatric Association (1994) Diagnosis and Statistical Manual of Mental Disorders. Washington DC, American Psychiatric Association.

Chapter 3

Developing community-based services and family support

3.1 The challenge of inclusion

Having a valued and respected place amongst a network of people and a rôle and inclusion in community life are important goals for all children and families. But challenging behaviour can create significant barriers to such community participation. Service providers and carers who work with children and families frequently comment on how they feel they are dealing with excluded or unwanted children.

The Committee heard of many instances of children and their families experiencing discrimination and exclusion both from services and from the community in general, thus denying them good quality child care and educational opportunities. It is almost impossible to overestimate these parents' anxiety and disappointment when their child was excluded or rejected in this way.

Concern was expressed that some local authorities were underestimating the complexity of children's needs. An overly simplistic understanding of inclusion meant that children were not always being offered the specialist inputs they needed in order to be able to use mainstream services. As a result, they were rapidly being excluded from such provision.

The Committee acknowledges that, in some instances, treatment or intervention in specialist and separate provision may be necessary to maximise the child's development and allow for a subsequent move to a less restrictive environment. However, 'special' and segregated services should always be part of a comprehensive programme of support, aimed at returning the child to their local communities with appropriate support at the earliest opportunity.

The Committee heard of families whose child was seen as 'too difficult' or 'too expensive' by local services providers:

'... we do resent what we feel to be silent derision or moral judgement if we, as parents, ask for an expensive service like a residential school. I was told that four children could be supported for the cost of what I was looking for. I said fine; it's feast or famine – the expensive 'gold star' service or nothing at all. I can't manage on nothing at all.' (A parent)

One parent suggested that better access to training and support for mainstream services would help to combat what she described as a 'crisis of competence and confidence' amongst staff, which could lead to children with complex needs being marginalised or rapidly excluded. Other parents felt that children with severe challenging behaviour were the victims of a lack of guidance for staff about issues such as the use of control and restraint. In some cases, the absence of a clear framework for tackling these issues provoked a fear of litigation resulting in children being excluded from integrated provision.

'No one is prepared to work together to see if they can cope. One teacher told me that the governors were really worried that if my child got aggressive, the school [a mainstream school with a unit attached] would be sued by other parents. They didn't feel they could take the risk. I had the same response from our local holiday playscheme. They said they would like to help, but they couldn't take the chance. The organiser said he felt all this passion for litigation was producing really negative outcomes, killing flexibility.' (A parent)

Of particular concern was the evidence we received about families who were only able to get help when they had reached breaking point. They can either struggle on or, as Donald's mother, reach the point where, without the support of local services, the only solution seems to be to request a residential placement and separation from her child.

'I can't even join a parents' support group because I think they wouldn't welcome Donald upsetting all their coffee mornings. Honestly, who would want us? I wouldn't if I was one of those parents. At Donald's next annual review I'm going to ask for a residential school placement. At least we'll get a break.'

Some parents spoke of being referred to 'Cinderella' services which, they felt, offered little or nothing more than containment of their child's difficulties. This was similar to the approach described in the Mansell Report (1993: 8) namely that adopted by the 'containers', who sought only to contain people in low-cost (and therefore poorly-staffed) settings.

This approach to service development and provision was in contrast to Mansell's 'developers' (DoH, 1993) who sought to provide local services which really do address individual needs and therefore give higher priority to funding services which, with more staff and more training and management input, are more expensive than ordinary community services.

3.2 The whole family

Each family will have its own particular coping mechanisms and its preferences and needs, yet the Committee heard of professionals who apparently 'knew' what was 'right' for families and what parents 'should' want:

'Try and understand what our family lives are really like.' (A parent)

'A whole family is affected by challenging behaviour.' (A parent)

When a child has challenging behaviour, the needs of families can get lost within the multiplicity of services involved in attempting to modify the child's behaviour (Quine, 1986, Peacock, Forrest and Mills, 1996). Treatments and other interventions may disrupt the home to the point where ordinary family life and the feelings and wishes of parents and other children are disregarded or marginalised.

'Seventy-four per cent [of carers] said their own needs had never been assessed. Fifty-one per cent of carers felt their needs were never taken into account and they were the 'unpaid and undervalued' work force that kept things together ... professionals kept going away.' (National Association of Carers, 1994)

Families placed considerable emphasis on the need for professionals to understand the whole family. They felt that the impact of severe challenging behaviour on siblings, particularly at critical times such as exams or school holidays, was not always recognised. The unacceptable behaviour of one child could also result in siblings being cut off from other young people so that they too had an impoverished social life.

Some families were concerned about the impact of the child's behaviour on their own personal relationships. One mother described how she and her husband 'divided up' the children between them, one taking the child with a learning disability, the other taking the siblings, to minimise disruption. She felt that no relationship could survive that degree of disruption.

Service providers may also ignore the fact that families are not static entities. Other family members may not always be around to help and support which is likely to have consequences for the level of formal support required. Siblings often give a great deal of help to a brother or sister with challenging behaviour, but they are also likely to leave home when they reach adulthood.

It is not only brothers and sisters who grow up, of course. The child with severe challenging behaviour moves through adolescence and into adulthood. There was widespread concern amongst parents about what would happen during and after this transition.

'[It's like] a dark abyss where we lose all our friends and trusted supporters and where young people can't have the same priority, when most local authorities are struggling with the increasing demands of a frail elderly population. The 'grey panthers' have votes but we don't. But really we need alliances, because we as parents are getting older too! Community care planning should take account of the prospective needs of children and young people, be pro-active not reactive and no one should have to 'jump' the hurdles at eighteen or nineteen or whenever someone thinks you have adult status.' (A parent)

Some parents pointed out that support services were not always aware of other responsibilities within the family and the impact this had on their ability to cope. Several parents of older children spoke of the 'double jeopardy' of intergenerational care where they were not only looking after a young person with severe challenging behaviour, but also caring for an elderly relative.

Patterns of family composition are changing all the time. There are many different types of 'family' and support services will have to be sufficiently flexible to adapt to very differing needs such as those of minority ethnic family groups and single-parent families. Socio-economic factors will also affect a family's ability to provide care for a child with complex needs. In particular the Committee was conscious that during its life-time, there was wide-spread debate about 'hard to reach' families, whose personal circumstances made it particularly difficult to access and use services. Although not receiving much direct evidence in this area, we were conscious of the multiple pressures on many families (for example, those coming from minority ethnic groups) and for services to be developed pro-actively and flexibly in order to meet their needs (Shah, 1996).

3.3 Family support

The term 'family support' has multiple meanings, encompassing both informal support and the more formal structured interventions offered by specialist services.

The Audit Commission (1994) defined family support as 'an activity or facility aimed at providing advice and support to parents to help them in bringing up children.' However, they also pointed to the very different interpretations of 'activities and facilities' and the resulting patchy and varied responses across the country.

The National Children's Bureau (1995) has proposed a fuller definition, based on the principle of 'community presence', which emphasises the importance of enabling families to access resources as and when they need them and to use their own skills to assist others.

'Family support is about the creation and enhancement, with and for families in need, of locally based (and accessible) activities, facilities and networks, the use of which will have outcomes such as alleviated stress, increased self-esteem, enhanced parental/carer/family competence and behaviour and increased parental/carer capacity to nurture and protect the children.' (National Children's Bureau, 1995)

Family support involves a delicate balancing act. Specialist support will usually be needed, but should always aim to support rather than supplant or undermine, parents' own coping abilities. The Leeds Early Education Support Network (Hearn, 1995) pointed out that parents could find it particularly difficult to balance the responsibility and decision-making which accompanies the care of all young children with specialist help. As they went on to say, being supportive, but allowing parents to keep control, is crucial if support and intervention are to be seen as positive and enabling.

The Committee also learned of a new approach being developed in the USA, where 'family preservation' aims to build up the confidence and competence of what are often seen as 'difficult' parents, so that they make better use of specialist services when necessary.

'The professionals and local people begin to work rather like an orchestra, each having their own special skills and specialist knowledge, but ... playing to the same tune as the supporting families, caring for children and enhancing community life.' (Hearn, 1995)

We believe that family support should be a key issue in local purchasing and commissioning arrangements and that any local arrangements for family support should be developed in active consultation with families with children with learning disabilities and severe challenging behaviour. As one parent succinctly pointed out:

'Many local authorities do consult with parents of children with learning disabilities. But their meetings and their methods of consultation may be impossible for families with children with severe challenging behaviour. We don't have the sitters or the short-term care to enable us to go to meetings. We are also often very tired. We can easily become a silent minority, unless there is a real commitment to find us and ask what we really need.'

3.4 Informal support

Fostering and supporting networks of informal care should be an essential component of any specialist service. This can reduce the possibility of social isolation or overdependence on professional assistance as well as helping ensure that any treatment or intervention programme has the maximum positive effect.

Family support must be everyone's business with informal support and specialist support services complementing and reinforcing one another in a positive fashion. Informal support is still too often ignored in professional debates about the nature of family support, when it should be seen as an integral part of it. As one parent pointed out, relatively low-key and informal community support systems and activities were often undervalued or not even known to specialist services, despite the fact that they often underpinned and made possible the more structured professional interventions.

Friends and neighbours, who welcome the child and other family members into their lives and perhaps offer occasional practical support, can really help to lessen the sense of isolation experienced by so many families. Informal support of this kind does not require professional skills or training, but it can and often does, have an important preventative function.

Positive acceptance of the child with challenging behaviour can enhance both the parents' and the child's self-esteem. It can give stressed or demoralised families much needed breathing space. But it can be more than simply preventative. Children can benefit by having access to a wider and richer range of activities and relationships which in turn can increase their self-confidence.

The importance of these kinds of informal supportive networks cannot be underestimated. Loneliness was a major problem for some families because their child's challenging behaviour placed limits on the whole family's social activities. Several parents stressed the value of informal community links; two families mentioning how their local church had made real efforts to include their children in activities.

3.5 Teamwork

The Committee heard of some families receiving confusing multiple services and others who had received inappropriate responses to requests for help with their child's challenging behaviour. In some instances, a lack of coordination made it difficult for families to access any help at all.

Opinions varied about who should coordinate treatment and other interventions. Some respondents felt strongly that a particular service should play a coordinating rôle: child development centres, child and adolescent mental health services, learning disability services and schools were all mentioned. Others felt that this should be the responsibility of particular professionals: clinical psychologists, psychiatrists specialising in children or learning disabilities and community paediatricians were suggested by various respondents.

Although there was no consensus about which option was preferable, there was general agreement that improved coordination within and between services was essential. However, whilst there was general agreement that specialist and generic children's services needed to work together more closely, in practice many services found such partnerships challenging.

A number of specific issues about teamwork were drawn to the Committee's attention:

▶ Some specialist staff were very isolated, reducing their ability to initiate and sustain a range of alternatives and leading to an unnecessarily limited range of interventions being offered to children and families.

▶ Specialist teams were often working directly with a child for a strictly limited period of time. If insufficient emphasis was placed on supporting services regularly used by that child, the effectiveness of specialist interventions was placed in jeopardy.

▶ Some services, which were strongly committed to inclusion and the use of mainstream services, were in danger of not accessing specialist services sufficiently early for interventions with challenging behaviour to be effective.

▶ Where staff in a particular service lacked knowledge and understanding of what other services had to offer, they could be reluctant to refer children and families to services which could be of real value to them.

One respondent to the Committee commented how child and adolescent mental health services are often misunderstood; because different services favour different approaches and may have little experience of alternative models of support and treatment, they may be very reluctant to agree to referrals at a sufficiently early point. Many challenging behaviours have escalated over a considerable period of time and greater understanding of reciprocal rôles and strengths would have facilitated better partnerships.

A properly coordinated, integrated teamwork approach was highly valued by parents. Children were sometimes referred to a range of services without any attempt at coherent planning to coordinate the various interventions. Parents also emphasised the importance of having an easily understood single point of access to treatment.

'Parents find it difficult to access services and to understand the different thresholds for assessment and access to particular provision.' (A parent)

Parents and other respondents suggested that the following characteristics would contribute to effective and coordinated services:

- An interdisciplinary and interactive style.
- A collaborative style of working which involved a wide range of professionals and carers.
- A dedicated and ring-fenced budget which enabled the service to adopt coherent approaches, develop specialisms and invest in enhancing the professional competence of staff.
- Effective leadership which encouraged opportunities for networking and shared learning opportunities with other specialist teams.
- A pro-active style of working which offered a service to children with 'inner-directed' behaviours such as depression or other mental health problems, as well as to those whose behaviour was outer-directed and therefore likely to challenge others.
- Staff with a high level of specialist knowledge, skills and expertise who offered competent and confident services, not only for diagnosis and assessment but also for maintenance of interventions in community settings.
- Specialist staff who were able to develop and sustain positive working relationships with staff in a wide range of community services in terms of initiating interventions and supporting their maintenance in those services.

Evidence from parents to the Committee endorsed the findings of other studies of families with children with severe disabilities (Baldwin and Carlisle, 1994; Beresford, 1995), demonstrating the isolation of many families; the stress caused by fragmented and poorly coordinated services and (as noted in Beresford, op cit) concerns that services often seemed to get fewer as children got older or if they had particularly complex special needs.

3.6 Parents as team members

The past decade has seen major changes in parental rôles. The 1996 Education Act and associated Code of Practice both envisage a greatly enhanced rôle for parents in terms of assessment and planning for meeting their child's special needs. In the voluntary sector we have seen the effectiveness of peer support and advice for potentially isolated and vulnerable families.

Within families too, some parents are providing 'hands-on' treatment for their children, sometimes (though not always) with professional support and supervision. (We define 'treatment' here as activities over and above the normal tasks and responsibilities of parenthood.) A number of recent evaluations of parental involvement in intervention programmes have demonstrated their effectiveness as therapists (Carpenter, 1995; Russell, 1995).

Active partnership with parents will always require a fine balance to be struck. Parents do not wish to be seen as a 'cheap resource', carrying out programmes for their child under the orders of professionals. But they do want to work in active partnership with professionals, to be involved in decisions about their child's treatment and perhaps undertake some interventions themselves. In particular, they want their views to be respected and given equal weight.

3.7 Short-term care

The past decade has seen major developments in the provision of short-term care for disabled children (Robinson, 1995; Stalker, 1995). The Committee was aware of the enormous value parents attached to good quality, regular short-term care. They were clear that the availability of local, flexible, child-centred respite services enabled them to continue caring for their child at home the rest of the time. As a national survey from the National Autistic Society indicated (Peacock, Forrest and Mills, 1996):

'parents of children with severely challenging behaviour can feel 'worn out and feeling utterly drained by the need for constant supervision without any end in sight' and 'the availability of appropriate services can make or break families with children with autism.'

On the other hand, we also heard about children using a number of different short-term care facilities, often at considerable distance from the family home. This seemed to stem from a lack of coherent planning or a full and proper consideration of how local support services might have enabled a child to remain in his or her local community.

Several parents commented that they had no option but to use whatever short-term care was offered even though this could mean leaving their child in a poor physical environment, with inadequately trained staff, a lack of personalised care and heavy reliance on medication. This is particularly worrying in the light of the proposed changes to the registration system for short-term care.

'Whatever I feel about my child's provision – I sit in the car and cry every time I leave him – I have to use respite care. Everybody out there talks about 'community' – well, they don't help with my child. No one wants him.' (A parent)

Children with severe challenging behaviour and learning disabilities can find it difficult to access family-based respite care. Parents felt their children were often excluded from family placement schemes because of their behavioural difficulties. Although the Norah Fry Research Centre (1995) found some schemes providing for children with challenging behaviour, they also found evidence that 'difficult' older children were often less easily placed.

The experiences of two families, each with a child with challenging behaviour and needing short-term care, demonstrate the very variable availability of this kind of support. Thomas's family have been unable to get the local authority to provide the respite care they need and are having to pay for a service which they know is not really appropriate. Although Thomas is supported in his own home, he lacks the opportunity to meet other children and make new relationships. Jeremy's family, on the other hand, are able to use a family placement scheme, despite his sometimes very challenging behaviour and respite is part of a well coordinated package of support.

'I got so desperate my grandmother said she'd pay for a break with a private care agency. I asked Age Concern for some local names. I thought they would know people who wouldn't be put off by behavioural difficulties [because of] dealing with dementia and all that. Really they were very good. I had a nurse coming every day and looking after Thomas. She did all sorts of things with him, but it cost nearly four hundred pounds a week. Of course, Thomas doesn't need nursing care, but who else will bother with him? I think it's really unfair that we should spend all that money on a break. I could have done with local authority funding and the money spent on a real holiday – or perhaps an extra staff member at a holiday play scheme.'

'We're really pleased with the help we've had for Jeremy .... Initially we couldn't get a family placement on the respite scheme; no one would consider Jeremy because he sometimes self-mutilates and he screams – really screams! But everyone got together and Jeremy's [respite] carer, ourselves and Jeremy's teacher all have a programme to work to.'

Foster families providing long-term care for children with learning disabilities and challenging behaviour will also need respite. One third of children in residential care have health or behaviour problems (OPCS, 1989) and a significant number of these will have been admitted following the breakdown of a family placement. Short-term breaks are important for all children with challenging behaviour and their carers, whether natural or substitute families.

Respite or short-term care is generally rather narrowly defined as 'sending the child somewhere else' (to another family, a residential care home or a hospital unit). Many families expressed the wish for a more flexible approach with the option of support in the home such as sitting services or day services. Some parents would like to hold their own short-term care budget which would enable them to pay other family members or friends, or au pairs. Not only is this likely to be more cost-effective but it would give parents a 'menu of options' for support at critical times.

3.8 Emergency care

The Committee heard from a number of parents about the importance of ensuring that emergency care is provided within the context of an overall policy on family support. Although well-planned short-term care can reduce demands for longer-term or permanent residential placement, parents need to be confident that their child will receive good quality and reliable care in a family emergency. Other relatives or neighbours are not usually able to provide substitute care for children with learning disabilities and challenging behaviour and volunteers frequently lack the kind of skills needed to support these children effectively.

Several parents (Council for Disabled Children, 1995) admitted having used long-stay hospital beds for emergency care for their older children. As one mother said: 'It's the one place where they always say yes.' She knew that National Health Service (NHS) provision was inappropriate for social care but pointed out that without any NHS input to local authority respite care, certain groups of children were frequently excluded from provision in the community.

If the child's main carer becomes ill, what may often be a rather fragile support system anyway is likely to fragment and collapse where the child has very challenging behaviour. The crisis may trigger further challenging behaviours if the child loses a sense of safety and security because their main care-giver is unavailable to them – perhaps in hospital.

Sefton Social Services Department (1995), which supports children with very challenging behaviour in the community, pointed out that an emergency service for vulnerable families may not always be fully utilised and funders must be prepared to meet the costs of what is essentially an 'insurance cover'.

We believe that respite services should be sufficiently flexible to be able to provide emergency cover.

Recommendations

Core recommendations

▶ Family support should be a key issue in local purchasing and commissioning arrangements which should acknowledge that some families will need a high degree of specialist support in order to continue to care for their child.

▶ The views and aspirations of families should inform all policy-making, planning and service development; consultation and participation arrangements need to recognise and be sensitive to the frequently heavy demands made on the time and energy of these families.

▶ The planning and provision of services should take into account the needs of the 'whole' family and the possible impact of any interventions on other family members such as siblings, particularly where interventions are home-based.

▶ Specialist services should seek to complement and reinforce informal support networks within local communities to reduce the potential isolation and marginalisation of families with a child with severe challenging behaviour.

Treatments and interventions

▶ Decisions about initiating home based treatments and interventions should always take account of the individual family's socio-cultural, economic and other circumstances.

▶ Parents should receive clear and accurate information to enable them to make informed choices about particular treatments and interventions. This information should include explanations about the nature and purpose of any proposed intervention, how it will be monitored and what the possible outcomes are.

▶ Decisions about treatments or other interventions which require a significant degree of parental involvement should only be made after parents have received clear and comprehensive information about the nature and the extent of their proposed rôle in any programme.

Short-term care

▶ Short-term care should be available within the context of a clear framework of assessment, care planning and review and should be an integral component of an individually planned support programme.

▶ A range of options should be available, including home-based respite such as sitting services or other domiciliary support, as well as family placements and other provision outside the home.

▶ Short-term care should be planned and provided in a sufficiently flexible manner to be able to respond to emergencies (eg parental illness) as well as offering planned (and where requested, regular) substitute care.

▶ The funding of short-term care should enable families to hold individual budgets if they so wish, so that they can purchase respite care when and from whom they wish, including friends, neighbours and other family members.

References

Audit Commission (1994) Seen but not Heard: Inter-Agency Collaboration in Services for Children in Need. HMSO.

Baldwin S and Carlisle J (1994) Social Support for Disabled Children and their Families: A Review of the Literature. HMSO.

Beresford B (1995) Expert Opinions: A National Survey of Parents Caring for Severely Disabled Children. Joseph Rowntree Foundation and Community Care.

Berridge D and Russell P (1993) – A Red Bus Next Time? Parents' Views of Special Educational Provision, Borough of Haringey. DFE.

Carpenter B (1994) Ed. Early Intervention: Where are we now? Oxford, Westminster Press.

Department of Health (1993) Services for People with Learning Disabilities and Challenging Behaviour or Mental Health Needs (Mansell Report). HMSO.

Hearn B (1995) Developing a Policy of Family Support. National Children's Bureau.

National Association of Carers (1994) Report of National Survey of Carers' Needs. National Association of Carers.

Office of Population and Census Surveys (1989) Disabled Children: Services Transport and Education. HMSO.

Peacock G Forrest A and Mills R (1996) Autism – the Invisible Children? An Agenda for Action. National Autistic Society.

Robinson C and Macadam M (1995) Balancing the Act: The Impact of the Children Act (1989) on Family Link Services for Children with Disabilities. Norah Fry Research Centre/Joseph Rowntree Foundation/National Children's Bureau.

Robinson C and Minkes J (1994) Assessing Quality in Services to Disabled Children under the Children Act (1989). Norah Fry Research Centre.

Russell P (1995) The Children Act (1989): Children and Young People with Learning Disabilities: Some Opportunities and Challenges. National Development Team.

Russell P (1995) Positive Choices: Services for Children with Disabilities Living Away from Home. Council for Disabled Children/National Children's Bureau.

Quine L and Pahl J (1985) Examining the causes of stress in families with severely mentally handicapped children. British Journal of Social Work, 15: 501-7.

Shah R (1996) The Silent Minority: Children with Disabilities in Asian Families. Second edition. National Children's Bureau.

Stalker K (1996) Ed. Developments in Short-term Care: Breaks and Opportunities. Research Highlights in Social Work, 25. Jessica Kingsley, Publishers.

CHAPTER 4: The rôle of education services

In considering the education of children and young people with learning disabilities and severe challenging behaviour, the Committee's starting point was that all children are entitled to a broad and balanced education as reflected in the spirit of the Code of Practice on the Identification and Assessment of Children with Special Educational Needs (DFE, 1994).

The Committee also wished to emphasise the central rôle played by the education service in the early identification of challenging behaviour and in the assessment, planning and review of any interventions. Evidence received clearly indicated the importance of partnership with schools, the educational psychology services and the local education authority (LEA) and the need for effective joint planning and implementation of any intervention programmes.

4.1 Background

In an educational setting, challenging behaviour will have particular implications for the child's full participation in the life of the school. Challenging behaviour may:

- prevent participation in educational activities;
- isolate children from their peer group and dramatically reduce opportunities for involvement in ordinary community activities;
- interfere with or affect the learning of other pupils;
- place the child or others in physical danger;
- make excessive demands upon teachers, staff and resources;
- make the possibilities for future placement problematic and increase the risk of exclusion.

Any discussion of the implications of challenging behaviour upon children's education must be put in the wider context of structural changes within the education system. The past few years have seen major changes in the organisation of education services in England and Wales, many of which affect children with special educational needs:

- The introduction of the National Curriculum for all pupils, though broadly welcomed by special schools, has imposed additional demands on them which can sometimes limit the time and resources available for working on a one-to-one basis with pupils with challenging behaviour.
- Increased parental choice in education means that schools, including special schools, face greater competition for pupils and are expected to demonstrate 'value for money' both to parents and to local education authorities (LEAs). This can lead to reluctance to admit pupils who are seen as having complex (and thereby expensive) special educational needs.
- Increased delegation of budgets to individual schools and pressure on resources in some LEAs may reduce their capacity to offer adequate and appropriate support and guidance to the most problematic children and to the schools they attend.
- An increasing emphasis on parental rights has led, in some instances, to children who display inappropriate behaviour being excluded from school as the result of pressure from parents of other pupils.
- There has been a significant increase in the number of exclusions of 'difficult' pupils from mainstream and special schools (including schools for pupils with severe learning disabilities).
- Growing concern amongst school staff and governing bodies about the legal basis for use of certain controls and treatments is leading some schools to exclude certain children because of ambivalence about permissible forms of control.

> 'With fewer resources available to the LEA to back us up in developing and managing behavioural and other programmes for our 'challenging' pupils, we have some hard decisions to make. How much of our budget should we allocate to such children? How skilled are our teachers to cope? INSET seems to be reducing too and in any event it is not the only thing we need.'
> (Head teacher, special school)

Other developments have been more specifically concerned with children with special educational needs:

- Implementation of Part III of the Education Act (1993) (now consolidated within the Education Act (1996)) and the Code of Practice (1994) so that assessments should now be carried out in clear stages, within defined timescales and with an emphasis on explicit target-setting, regular reviews and parental involvement.
- The introduction of the Special Educational Needs Tribunal, allowing for independent appeals against LEA decisions.
- Publication of the government's Pupils with Problems circulars, notably Circular No. 2 (DFE, 1993).
- A requirement (in the Code of Practice) for all schools, including special schools to draw up policies on special educational needs which must be reviewed annually and which are scrutinised as part of the OFSTED inspection process. This emphasises the enhanced responsibility which individual schools are expected to assume for identifying, assessing and meeting a range of special educational needs.

4.2 Definitions

As already noted in Chapter 2, there are many different and sometimes overlapping terms used to define children with special needs including 'learning disability' (commonly used in health and social services).

The Committee was concerned that there was evidence of some confusion amongst purchasers and providers about children with 'emotional and behavioural difficulties' and those with 'challenging behaviour'. Although the two definitions can overlap, we wish to emphasise again the importance of clear definitions.

4.3 Early intervention

As already noted, the importance of effective early identification and intervention to address challenging behaviour, before it becomes well established, cannot be underestimated. Pre-school education services and schools have a key rôle to play in this respect; they are often the principal or only setting where a child's behaviours can be consistently observed outside the family setting.

The Committee heard some concerns expressed about changes in the organisation of nursery education. There was particular concern about the introduction of the voucher scheme which is likely to result in an increasingly diversified and de-regulated marketplace for pre-school education following full implementation of the scheme from November 1996. One consequence of these changes has been increasingly common practice in many LEAs of admitting 'rising four year olds' to full-time primary education. This trend has particular significance for children with learning disabilities and challenging behaviour, for whom two years in nursery education offer important opportunities for personal as well as educational development. Many of these children would not be easily included within a primary school curriculum at the proposed earlier age of full time school entry.

Although there are currently few evidence-based early intervention programmes of proven benefit to the cognitive development or the longer term management of behaviour in the child, evaluations of Portage and other home based learning programmes show considerable benefit to parents, through improving their self confidence and their ability and willingness to continue to work with very challenging children.

4.4 A 'whole school' approach

> 'Parent power is now an issue in special schools too. By 'parent power' I mean that parents may complain to governors if they think that certain children put their own children at risk because of their behaviour or if they feel their children's education is very disrupted. I feel ... that everybody in

a school has to own the issue of pupils with difficult behaviour. If there is no common ownership of the problem (and its solution) then exclusions will continue to rise in special schools too.'
(Head teacher, special school)

From evidence we received, it is clear that implementing particular strategies around individual children with challenging behaviour is more likely to be effective if they are part of a school's overall approach to supporting children with special needs. Key issues to be addressed included:

▶ **Resource management:** The creative deployment of all the school's resources in support of the learning of all its pupils (including agreement about how the school proposes to allocate its learning support budget) and an awareness of other resources outside the school which might be accessed (eg child and adolescent mental health services).

▶ **Professional staff development:** An active commitment to developing the skills and expertise of all staff in ways that enable the school to respond in a positive fashion to the diverse needs of its pupils. This would include use of INSET opportunities, local and national training opportunities (including distance learning), support from other professionals and joint working and skills-sharing with other services.

▶ **Collaborative working:** A recognition that supporting and helping children with challenging behaviour should not be the sole responsibility of one member of staff or even one department. This means developing 'whole school' policies for the management of difficult behaviours so that everyone can respond positively to the challenge.

'The South Glamorgan Challenging Behaviour Service is jointly managed by education and social services. It is able to provide a range of individualised supports to children with a range of challenging behaviours and emotional and behavioural difficulties. The Service works with parents, teachers and children, on a one-to-one basis if necessary to develop and maintain strategies to support children within school and to manage challenging behaviour as effectively as possible and to facilitate a return to community services after exclusion where this has occurred.'

▶ **Special educational needs policies:** The importance of including specific reference to the management of challenging behaviour and prioritising resources in order to address the needs of children with complex difficulties.

4.5 Responding to children with severe learning disabilities who present challenging behaviour

In taking evidence on how schools might respond most effectively to children with challenging behaviour, the Committee drew upon recent research by John Harris (Chief Executive, BILD) and colleagues (Harris et al, 1996) which looked at the experiences of 44 special schools for pupils with severe learning disabilities in the West Midlands. The Committee was also able to take evidence from special residential schools with a particular expertise in the management of the most challenging behaviours.

Respondents listed a range of behaviours in school settings which were particularly problematic for staff including:

▶ physical aggression;
▶ self injury;
▶ shouting, swearing, loud noises;
▶ distractibility and hyperactivity;
▶ obsessional and ritualistic behaviour;
▶ non compliance and resistance to teaching, with disruptive behaviour which also interfered with other children's learning.

In developing strategic responses to these and other challenging behaviours, a number of positive responses and interventions were noted. These included:

4.5.1 Helping pupils to develop positive relationships

Many pupils with challenging behaviour experience considerable difficulty in forming relationships. In consequence they may be presumed to be indifferent to other people and unaffected by placement with a number of different adults each day. This approach may be helpful to teachers who can share the demands which arise from challenging behaviour. However, this Committee considers that many children who challenge need opportunities in school to develop a relationship with one adult so that they can acquire the basic skills for social interaction and communication.

4.5.2 The need to focus on teaching language and communication

The Committee accepted that many different factors contribute to challenging behaviours and that for any single behaviour, multiple causation is likely to be the rule rather than the exception. However, there is a growing body of evidence (Harris et al, 1993 and Harris, 1994) to suggest that problems with communication may play a significant part in the emergence of some challenging behaviours. For example, a significant number of children who present challenging behaviours also have delayed language development (Kiernan and Kiernan, 1994) and other studies suggest that challenging behaviour can be reduced by teaching pupils communicative behaviours which attract appropriate responses from teachers and carers (Durand, 1990). In effect, pupils need to experience the power of communication in ordinary everyday settings where it can help them to express their own feelings and meet their own needs (Harris, 1994, 1996).

4.5.3 Planning activities to match pupils' strengths and weaknesses

A number of respondents told the Committee of their concern at the increasing emphasis on structured teaching situations in special schools in order to meet the requirements of the National Curriculum. This could cause problems for pupils with severe challenging behaviour because of:

- their very limited concentration which meant they were unable to work successfully with other pupils;
- their narrow range of interests which may shade into obsessive preoccupations;
- their very different levels of ability in comparison with their peers.

Challenging behaviour may also make the assessment of levels of ability, interests and attention spans very problematic. However, we were also aware that some schools are developing individualised and differentiated programmes of work which reflect the ability and interests of children with challenging behaviour.

4.5.4 Ensure that all staff are aware of new methods of work

New methods of working with pupils with challenging behaviours will be ineffective unless they are introduced consistently throughout the school and all members of staff are briefed and fully prepared to implement new approaches. The Committee identified a number of potential barriers to integrated approaches within schools including:

- wide variations in the formal training of staff;
- inconsistent responses to challenging behaviours by individual teaching and non-teaching staff in the school;
- few schools with effective strategies for disseminating new ways of working with individual pupils to staff throughout the school.

Some schools already had, or were in the process of establishing, written protocols or management plans setting out how they would respond to particular behaviours. These could serve as a fixed point of reference against which staff could monitor whether their own and their colleagues' performance lay in line with the protocol or management plan.

Harris (1995) notes that whilst many staff currently make written plans for their curriculum-based work, it seems likely that further support material and training will be needed if a similarly rigorous approach is to be widely used as part of a response to challenging behaviour.

It was clear to the Committee that some schools have developed effective strategies which can be integrated within current educational practice. But the Committee was concerned to narrow the divide which often exists between clinical expertise being developed outside schools and school based responses to pupils who present challenging behaviour.

4.6 Children with emotional and behavioural difficulties

Although the Committee made a clear distinction between children with emotional and behavioural difficulties (but without a learning disability) and children with learning disabilities and severe challenging behaviour, it was taking evidence during a period of intense public interest and debate about 'difficult and disruptive pupils'. The Committee was also aware that some children with learning disabilities and severe challenging behaviour would also experience disadvantage and deprivation, abuse or poor parenting which would exacerbate their behaviours and inhibit the effective implementation of any intervention strategies if not acknowledged.

Therefore, although the government Circular 'On the education of children with emotional and behavioural difficulties' (DFE 1993) does not deal specifically with children with learning disabilities and challenging behaviour, several respondents pointed out its relevance and usefulness in relation to this group. They suggested that lessons could be learned from some of the innovative work being carried out with children with emotional and behavioural difficulties and that more networking, joint working, shared training and pooling knowledge and experience would be helpful.

Three key issues emerge regarding the development of appropriate educational responses to address the needs of children with challenging behaviour and children with emotional and behavioural difficulties:

▶ the importance of early identification of behavioural problems so that specialist advice can be sought where necessary;

▶ the need for early and effective liaison between education, social services and child health services when planning provision; and

▶ the use of controls and sanctions (see Chapter 7).

Under the terms of the Circular, every school must have a written policy on the management of pupils' behaviour. This must include:

▶ confirmation of each child's entitlement to a broadly-based curriculum, including National Curriculum and religious education;

▶ the rewards and sanctions to be used in helping young people learn how to behave acceptably;

▶ detailed procedures to be followed where behaviour is extreme including recording specific behaviour causing concern, staff responses and the outcomes;

▶ confirmation that the young person will be involved as fully as possible in agreeing behaviour management programmes;

▶ clear arrangements for regular monitoring, evaluation and review of behaviour management programmes;

▶ acknowledgement that staff must be familiar with a range of behaviour management approaches so they can select the most appropriate intervention in response to a child's particular need and, through training, be skilled in the application of such approaches.

The circular also emphasises the importance of staff involved with behaviour management regimes being regularly and properly supervised to safeguard against potential abuse.

Section 26 of the Education Bill, which was going through Parliament as this report went to press, will require LEAs to develop and publish up-to-date policies and plans for dealing with all pupils with behaviour problems. Schools will also be required to have behaviour policies (which should complement the existing requirement to have policies on special educational needs). Such policies must set out both the arrangements within school and any arrangements made if the child is excluded and requires provision outside the school at which he or she is a pupil.

4.7 Exclusions of pupils with challenging behaviour

The Education Act (1993) (now the 1996 Act) and the 'Pupils with Problems' circulars set out a framework for the management of exclusions of pupils from school and the arrangements to be made following exclusions. During the Committee's life time, the number of pupils excluded from school escalated sharply. Although the majority of these were not exclusions from special schools, the Committee was concerned to learn that exclusions from special schools were part of this overall increase.

This was confirmed by the findings of Christ Church College, Canterbury (1996) which showed that the total number of exclusions rose by eight per cent during 1995-96 and also a worrying trend of increasing numbers of pupils excluded from special schools. Christ Church College found that many of these excluded children received only minimal alternative education provision and frequently had difficulty finding another school. In an increasingly performance-linked climate, he also found that school governors were under pressure to exclude more often than had hitherto been the case.

A head teacher, writing to the Committee, commented:

'I am increasingly concerned by growing evidence of actual or attempted exclusions of children with challenging behaviour from special schools. The reasons for this trend are manifold. First, the pattern of childhood disability is changing. Our new intake [in an SLD school] contains far more children who are 'medically frail'. They have multiple and profound disabilities and the presence of an active and potentially aggressive child can be a real challenge. Our governors (we are now a grant maintained school) and the parents' organisation see this group of [medically frail] children as increasing and our main priority. The more able children who might once have come here are either in MLD schools or units or even in mainstream schools. I should add that the situation is made worse by budget pressures and staff cuts. If the classroom assistant is off sick, then we cannot cope with a child with challenging behaviour.' (Personal communication)

These concerns were echoed in other evidence to the Committee. Although we were not able to identify the exact numbers of pupils with learning disabilities and severe challenging behaviour currently excluded from school nor the reasons for exclusions, we did receive evidence of:

▶ the changing population of many special schools, with more severely and multiply disabled pupils whose needs were incompatible with very active or challenging children;

▶ the increasing reduction in LEA central support services, because of delegation of budgets;

▶ pressure on school budgets generally, with larger classes even within special schools and reductions in the availability of trained non-teaching assistants;

▶ pressure from other parents, who were anxious about their children being injured or distracted by children with very challenging behaviour;

▶ pressure on LEAs to divert resources to statutory assessment and statements. (Between 1985 and 1996, the number of statements rose from 128,000 to 229,000. (DfEE, 1996)) The educational psychology service in particular described itself as overstretched, with LEAs also having to invest resources in the new arrangements for statutory annual reviews and transition plans.

In addition to these pressures on schools and LEAs, the Committee also heard from families about how exclusion could affect their lives including family breakdown and/or the child's removal into residential care.

4.8 Residential education

'Some seriously disturbed children pass through many community and school-based forms of provision and arrive in residential accommodation only after further damage is inflicted by multiple rejections and failures. It is then often too late for the schools concerned to achieve positive change. Made at the right time, residential placements can be a positive option.' (DFE, Circular 9/94)

Evidence received by the Committee emphasised the importance of early identification and intervention in preventing or ameliorating challenging behaviours, but also acknowledged that residential education can be a positive option when children need the very specialist help which can only be provided within a residential setting. However, the Committee was concerned at the apparent lack of clear criteria for the placement of some children with challenging behaviour and the corresponding absence of clear targets and regular review arrangements. The Committee heard of crisis admissions to residential education, with pressure from some social services departments for schools to offer 52 weeks a year care. Two residential schools also reported that arrangements for returning a pupil to a local school could be problematic and that local authorities were less willing to invest in maintenance arrangements when the child returned home than in the initial crisis placement.

Several residential schools referred to the timescale and difficulties in agreeing funding arrangements for placements when such a placement was expected to provide a mix of educational, social, medical or mental health support. Although some LEAs had panels or forums through which joint funding arrangements could be negotiated prior to any placement decision, the majority did not.

One LEA expressed particular concern about future patterns of provision for children with 'low incidence' disabilities (in particular, challenging behaviour). They pointed to the lack of expertise about such disabilities in many of the new unitary authorities and the absence of criteria for determining 'value for money' in any special provision.

4.9 Parent participation

The Committee was aware that the introduction of the Code of Practice, together with development of the rôle of the 'named person' through parent partnership schemes, provided a new framework for the active involvement of parents within their children's education. In practice, parental responses were variable. Some parents were very positive about their rôle in developing, implementing and reviewing individual programmes. They felt that their concerns were taken seriously and that their children were making progress. Other parents felt that they were insufficiently involved; that home school liaison was not always as effective as it could be and that their children's behaviour made their position in the school very vulnerable.

Parents whose children had experienced a late diagnosis (in particular parents of autistic children) felt that valuable time had been lost by delays in making a diagnosis and were the most likely to feel that the school lacked specialist expertise. Some parents had actively chosen specialist residential schools and were very positive about the integration of education and social care and about the range of educational options available.

Parental perceptions of assessment and participation in school-based activities will vary according to individual expectations and the organisation of the school in question. However, an OFSTED report (1996) on the first three years of implementation of the Code of Practice clearly indicated wide variations in policy and practice in schools with regard to partnership with parents. All schools (including special schools) are required to have school special educational needs policies and OFSTED's conclusions bears out evidence to the Committee, namely that partnership arrangements were highly variable in terms of their quality and coherence.

Recommendations

Definitions

▶ All purchasers and providers should familiarise themselves with the Code of Practice (DFE, 1994), the Pupils with Problems circulars and their local LEA's relevant policies to ensure that referrals and interventions are appropriate, timely and based upon mutually agreed and clear definitions of a child's learning disability and severe challenging behaviour and any related special educational or other needs.

Early identification and intervention

▶ LEAs should have the necessary procedures in place to ensure that any behavioural difficulties are identified without delay so that appropriate referrals and potential interventions can be considered.

▶ Nursery schools and classes and other providers of pre-school provision should receive appropriate advice and support from their local educational psychology service in order to support young children with learning disabilities and severe challenging behaviour. This should include addressing the training and support needs of pre-school teaching and non-teaching staff.

▶ The Department for Education and Employment (DfEE) should actively promote home-based learning programmes (and Portage in particular).

▶ The DoH, together with the DfEE should invest in research programmes to evaluate the effectiveness of the range of early interventions so that purchasers and commissioners have clearer outcomes measures on which to base their decision.

Management of challenging behaviour

▶ The DfEE must consider urgently the training and development needs of teaching and ancillary staff working with pupils with severe challenging behaviour.

▶ Effective classroom strategies for working with pupils with severe challenging behaviour which can be validated in terms of developmental theory should be more widely disseminated and further research undertaken into the small number of pupils whose behaviour is not ameliorated or halted by any current interventions.

Curriculum and policies

▶ The School Curriculum and Assessment Authority (SCAA) should, as a matter of urgency, address the curricular needs of children with learning disabilities and severe challenging behaviour and, in particular, address the need to acquire and record Level 1 skills which are not part of the National Curriculum framework.

▶ The requirement under the Education Act 1996 and the Code of Practice that every school (including special schools) must draw up a policy on special educational needs should include a specific reference as to how the school proposes to meet the needs of children with learning disabilities and severe challenging behaviour.

▶ The current Education Bill (1996) requiring LEAs to produce behaviour management policies should complement and reinforce the special educational needs policies referred to above. Behaviour management policies should include clear information about alternative provision to be made for any children who may be at risk of exclusion.

Exclusions

▶ The DfEE should require LEAs to collect data on exclusions which would enable them to identify the numbers of pupils with learning disabilities and severe challenging behaviour who are being excluded, the reasons for their exclusion and the alternative provision made for the child.

Parent participation

▶ The DfEE should, through LEAs, very actively encourage all schools and particularly special schools, to spell out clearly within their special needs policies, the arrangements for involving parents in assessment, development of individual programmes and reviews. Policies should also specify what information is given to parents and ways in which the school can give particular support to vulnerable parents.

▶ LEAs and schools should ensure that all parents receive information about local and national voluntary organisations which may be able to offer advice and information and the telephone number of the local Parent Partnership Officer, to ensure that they have access to independent advice and representation if required. Because of the potential isolation of many parents of children with learning disabilities and severe challenging behaviour, LEAs should work with the local voluntary sector and Parent Partnership Scheme to review regularly and update the information, advice and representation offered to parents of children with learning disabilities and severe challenging behaviour during assessment and review.

References

Canterbury Christ Church College (1996) Final Report to the Department for Education: National survey of local education authorities' policies and procedures for the identification of and provision for children who are out of school by reason of exclusion or otherwise. Canterbury, Christ Church College.

Department of Education (1993) The Education of Children with Emotional and Behavioural Difficulties Pupils with Problems Circular No 2. DFE.

DFE (1994) Code of Practice on the Identification and Assessment of Special Educational Needs. DFE.

DFE (1994) Education of Children with Emotional and Behavioural Difficulties. DFE Circular 9/94.

DfEE (1996) Nursery Education Voucher Scheme: The Guide. DfEE.

DfEE (1996) Code of Practice on the Identification and Assessment of Special Educational Needs: Nursery Education Voucher Scheme: Guidance on the Application of the Code to institutions outside the maintained sector of education who wish to redeem nursery education vouchers. DfEE.

Department of Health/DfEE (1996) Children's Services Planning Guidance Inter-agency Working Users and Children in Need.

Durand V and Crimmins D (1991) Teaching functionally equivalent responses as an intervention for challenging behaviour. In: The Challenge of Severe Mental Handicap: A Behaviour Analytical Approach. Ed. B Remington. John Wiley and Sons.

Felce D and McBrien J (1992) Working with People who have Severe Learning Difficulty and Challenging Behaviour: A Practical Handbook on the Behavioural Approach. British Institute of Learning Disabilities.

Harris J (1994) Language communication and personal power a developmental perspective. Ed. J Couple 0'Kane and B Smith Taking Control Enabling People with Learning Difficulties. David Fulton Publishers.

Harris J Cook M and Upton G (1993) Challenging behaviour in the classroom. In: Innovations in Education with Children with Severe Learning Difficulties. Ed. J Harris. Lisieux Hall.

Harris J (1995) Responding to pupils with severe learning disabilities who present challenging behaviour. British Journal of Special Education 22, 3: 109-115.

Harris J and Cook M (1995) A Whole School Approach to Working With Pupils With Severe Learning Difficulties and Challenging Behaviour. British Institute of Learning Disabilities Publication (workshop training materials).

Harris J Cook M and Upton G (1996) Pupils with Severe Learning Disabilities who Present Challenging Behaviour: A Whole School Approach to Assessment and Intervention. British Institute of Learning Disabilities Publication.

Kiernan C and Kiernan D (1994) Challenging Behaviour in Schools for Pupils with Severe Learning Difficulties. Mental Handicap Research 7: 117-201.

OFSTED (1996) The Implementation of the Code of Practice OFSTED.

Quine (1985) Examining the causes of stress in families with severely mentally handicapped children. British Journal of Social Work, 15: 501-7.

Sylva K (1996) Evaluation of the High Scope Programme. Oxford University Press.

CHAPTER 5
Away from home: residential provision

5.1 Introduction

The Committee received only limited evidence about children with learning disabilities and severe challenging behaviour who were living apart from their families on a long-term basis. However, our general impression is that they were more likely to be placed outside their local community than children without significant behaviour problems.

We are extremely concerned about the isolation and consequent vulnerability of these young people, an increasing number of whom are in residential establishments for fifty-two weeks a year. Perhaps this lack of evidence reflects their isolated situation.

Children with learning disabilities and challenging behaviour may be living in one of the following types of residential setting:

▶ residential schools (up to 52 weeks a year);
▶ specialist residential homes;
▶ NHS facilities (eg specialist units);
▶ secure accommodation.

Although the decision to admit a child to a residential setting may be in that child's best interests and may be the most appropriate solution for a particular individual, the Committee is aware that too often such decisions are reactive, made in response to a crisis. A child's placement may well be determined by the availability, regardless of whether it is the most appropriate option.

5.2 Criteria for use of residential provision

There was overwhelming agreement by the Committee that wherever possible children should be cared for at home or in locally-based services. We recognise this will require a significant expansion of local services, including the use of ordinary houses in ordinary streets. Residential services do not necessarily have to involve out-of-area placements, although at present they often do.

But we also recognise that a small number of children have special needs which at present cannot be safely or adequately addressed within local services. They need the type of care, treatment or education which currently can only be provided within a specialist residential setting.

Admitting a child with challenging behaviour to residential provision should:

▶ be a positive, pro-active choice (eg to halt escalation of challenging behaviour by carrying out an assessment and setting up treatment programme). In other words, the residential provision should have something positive to offer the child and family;

▶ be the most appropriate form of provision, eg children who do not require any specific medical interventions should not be placed in hospital or in other NHS facilities;

▶ not be seen as a permanent solution; interventions should be aimed at helping the child return to his or her local community.

[Children may] 'arrive in residential accommodation only after further damage is inflicted by multiple rejections and failures. It is then often too late for the schools concerned to achieve significant change. Made at the right time, residential placement can be a positive option' (DfEE, Circular 9/94)

'Lucy's parents initially felt it was a real failure for their daughter to attend a residential special school – until they realised that for Lucy, the 'least restrictive environment' was a special one where she felt safe and where she could be helped.' (Teacher)

5.3 Current use of residential provision

Admissions to long-term residential provision occur for a number of reasons. These may have to do with the child. For example:

- escalation of challenging behaviour;
- onset of acute mental illness;
- law-breaking activities;
- a need for specialist (medical) investigation.

Residential placement may also be the result of:

- the child's family no longer being able to provide care;
- breakdown of a placement with a substitute family;
- lack of regular and appropriate short-term respite care;
- an emergency within the child's family, eg the primary care giver becomes seriously ill;
- local community services no longer being able to provide care;
- closure of local residential facilities without replacement by appropriate local alternatives.

The need for a residential placement will often be related to a combination of these factors, eg the child's challenging behaviour escalates because of other difficulties within the family; or a young person's exclusion from local services leads to a request by the family for long-term residential care. However, we were aware of an encouraging concern across children's services to make decisions about residential placements on the basis of clear and agreed local criteria such as those set out by the DFE (1994) in Circular 9/94 and some local initiatives through inter-agency planning to work collaboratively in planning, funding and reviewing any placements.

Evidence from parents and parent-led organisations suggests that some families are 'choosing' longer-term residential options if they are unable to access flexible short-term care as and when needed.

'Parents need practical daily support when they are caring for a child with very difficult behaviour. They need help before they break down …. If things don't get better we will be looking for a residential placement. At least it would keep us together.' (A parent)

The Committee believes that if purchasers and commissioners were to prioritise the development of good quality preventive services, including appropriate early intervention, future demand for more expensive out-of-area placements could be considerably reduced.

5.4 Residential provision and collaboration

The use of residential provision – whether in a hospital, school or secure unit – has a number of potential disadvantages:

- the setting may be a long way from the child's family home;
- provision may be in a very rural setting, isolated from normal patterns of community life;
- the use of out-of-area services may be a disincentive to local services developing the necessary skills and competence to work with children with challenging behaviour;
- there is greater potential for children being subject to abuse where they are separated from their families;
- staff in isolated, sometimes small-scale, residential services may be more in danger of burn out than those working in community-based services.

The Committee believes that to ameliorate or overcome these potential difficulties, residential services need to develop and maintain active links with families and with local services in the communities to which these children belong – and to which, hopefully, they will return.

Children and their families should be encouraged to maintain contact with one another in ways which are most appropriate and practicable for the child and the family concerned. Any or all of the following could be used – visits, telephone calls, letters, audio tapes and videos. The appointment of an Independent Visitor (The Children Act (1989)) may be helpful when the child is at a considerable distance from the family home or when family contact is problematic.

The recently revised action and assessment materials for children 'looked after' by the local authority (Ward, 1995, DoH, 1995) can help to ensure that an holistic assessment of the child's health, social care, personal and educational needs is carried out. This should enable an informed decision to be made and one which is in the child's best interests, particularly when a residential placement may be planned primarily because of family difficulties in caring for the child in the family home.

5.5 Secure accommodation

'The government should, as a matter of urgency, convene a major review of all law and policy ... relating to the locking up of children, with a view to securing the aim of Article 37 of the UN Convention on the Rights of the Child – that the child should be locked up only as a last resort and for the shortest appropriate time (National Children's Bureau, 1995) ... restricting the liberty of children is a serious step which must be taken only when there is no appropriate alternative. It must be a last resort in the sense that all else must first have been considered comprehensively and rejected – never because no other placement was available at the relevant time or because of inadequacies in staffing.' (DoH, 1995)

Information on the type of behaviours which lead to the placement of individual young people in secure accommodation is currently unavailable. But despite this, the Committee decided it must consider the use of secure accommodation, not least because of a growing concern about the circumstances of people with learning disabilities within the penal system.

Furthermore, although the total number of children with learning disabilities and challenging behaviour in secure units is probably relatively small, their situation has wider relevance. It highlights the importance of using specialist residential provision only when it has something positive to offer a child, rather than as a last resort when more appropriate services are not available.

There is growing concern that a number of children with learning disabilities and severe behaviour disorders are being placed in secure units because of lack of appropriate alternatives. There is also evidence – albeit largely anecdotal – that some young people with learning disabilities and severe challenging behaviour may be at risk of offending and thus particularly vulnerable to placement in secure units.

5.6 The legal basis for use of secure accommodation

Under s25 the Children Act (1989), children being looked after by the local authority may be placed in secure (ie locked) accommodation for one or more of the following reasons:

▶ they have a history of 'absconding', are likely to abscond from other accommodation and in doing so are likely to suffer 'significant harm';

▶ they might injure themselves or others if in other accommodation.

Several organisations and individuals have pointed to the impact of the rapid expansion of secure accommodation. Harris and Timms (1992), for example, who undertook research on behalf of the DoH have commented that:

'the most important predictor of the high usage of secure accommodation is a local authority's possession of a secure unit.'

Their views have been echoed by others:

'the additional places [in secure accommodation] were rapidly filled ... we are still ... wondering how it is possible to provide more secure accommodation without it being filled with children who do not need to be there.' (National Association of Guardians ad Litem and Reporting Officers, 1992).

'The use of secure accommodation tends to reflect the availability of places rather than careful consideration of the contribution of such accommodation ... [it] may therefore bridge a gap in appropriate community services rather than offer something discrete and significant in managing a child's very difficult behaviour.' (National Children's Bureau, 1995).

In a recent national survey (Hodgkin, 1995), managers of secure units considered that 60 out of 193 children in their care could have been safely placed in open accommodation. Despite the DoH guidance (1995) quoted above, it appears that these children are only in secure units because more suitable alternatives in the community do not exist.

5.7 The impact of privatisation

Commenting on the possible effects of 'privatising' secure accommodation (Hodgkin, 1995), managers of secure units have expressed concern that financial considerations could lead to units being run on the 'hotel' principle (eg minimising vacancies), so that any child is accepted regardless of whether the unit is the most appropriate provider of care for that child or whether the placement is compatible with the needs of other residents.

Recommendations

Criteria for the use of residential provision

▶ Residential provision should only be considered after non-residential options have been carefully considered and excluded, as either not being in the child's best interests or as being unable to meet the child's current needs.

▶ Purchasers in health, education and social services should agree clear criteria for using residential provision, which should be seen as a positive option, rather than as a stop-gap because of the inadequacy of other services.

▶ The decision to use residential provision should be based on a comprehensive multi-disciplinary assessment, following which a child care plan should be agreed, setting out short-term targets, longer term objectives and arrangements for regular review agreed. The recently revised assessment, action and review materials for children 'looked after' by the local authority (DoH, 1995) provide a model for an holistic assessment of the child's health, social care, personal and educational needs.

▶ Where a child is admitted to a residential service on an emergency basis, a full assessment should be completed within a maximum period of six months and should include full consideration of the reasons for admission.

▶ In the case of an out-of-area placement the purchaser-provider contract should specify how the child will be enabled to return to his or her local community and how the family and community services will be assisted to support the child after returning home.

NHS Provision

▶ Facilities for in-patient assessment, diagnosis and treatment should be available if required. This may necessitate an expansion of specialist facilities. Such facilities should include out-reach support for staff working in community based services, including educational provision, to enhance their confidence and competence in working with children with learning disabilities and severe challenging behaviour within local services wherever possible.

▶ Health authority purchasing and commissioning arrangements should prioritise the development of good quality preventive services and ensure that children with learning disabilities and severe challenging behaviour have equality of access to specialist diagnostic facilities.

Liaison with families and coordination between services

▶ Staff in all residential services should liaise regularly with families to discuss their child's progress, keep them informed about treatments and other interventions and consider plans for the future. Depending on individual circumstances, such liaison could be via meetings, written communications and telephone calls. Every effort should be made to ensure that parents are actively involved in any assessments or reviews. Where necessary assistance with travel costs and child-care for other children should be made available.

▶ Staff in residential services should work with local services to offer guidance, support and back-up in helping families and community services to feel able to care for children and manage their behaviour when they return home. Joint planning by residential and community services should begin well in advance of the child leaving residential care. Parents should be closely involved in any planning arrangements for a child's return home.

▶ Where a child in residential accommodation has little or no family contact, an Independent Visitor (the Children Act (1989)) should be appointed to encourage family links and help safeguard the child's interests through offering independent advocacy and support.

▶ A range of residential provision should be developed, including: ordinary houses in residential areas; residential schools with outreach services linked to children's families and communities; specialist psychiatric beds with associated outreach services; and specialist neuropsychiatric beds [for assessment and diagnosis]. All services should be available from the possible residential options within [and outside] their communities.

Secure accommodation

▶ The DoH should monitor the placement of and issue clear guidelines on the criteria for admitting young people with learning disabilities and severe challenging behaviour to secure accommodation.

▶ Local strategic planning, including Children's Services Plans, together with joint purchasing and commissioning arrangements, should specify the arrangements they propose to make to support children at risk of admission to secure provision as well as services for those leaving secure accommodation.

▶ Health services, (particularly child and adolescent mental health services), social services, LEA and criminal justice agencies should work closely together to ensure an integrated approach to assessment and treatment so that secure provision is not used solely for purposes of 'containment'.

References

Department of Education (1994) The Education of Children with Emotional and Behavioural Difficulties, Circular 9/94 Pupils with Problems. DFE.

Department of Health (1995) Looking after Children Training Resources Pack. HMSO.

Hodgkin R (1995) Safe to Let Out? The Current and Future Use of Secure Accommodation. National Children's Bureau.

Russell P (1995) Positive Choices: Services for Children with Disabilities Living Away from Home. Council for Disabled Children/National Children's Bureau.

Ward H (1995) Ed. Looking after Children Research into Practice: Second Report to the DoH on Assessing Outcomes in Child Care. HMSO.

Utting W (1991) Children in Public Care. HMSO.

CHAPTER 6 Treatments

6.1 Introduction

When considering the wide range of evidence the Committee received, a series of issues concerning the treatment of children with learning disabilities and severe challenging behaviour emerged, which the Committee decided needed to be addressed.

The term 'treatment' is used here to describe specific interventions that are intended to prevent, ameliorate, cure or reduce the frequency of challenging behaviour once the behaviour is apparent. It does not refer only to medical treatment but refers to psychological, environmental, psycho-therapeutic and 'alternative' treatments.

The Committee was aware that for children with severe challenging behaviour, their problems tend to be complex and to persist over time. Different approaches may need to be tried and regular review is essential. We have used evidence of effectiveness where this is available. The Committee is aware that some parents or children may prefer particular sorts of treatment and find others unacceptable or intrusive. In deciding how to facilitate choice and ensure that effective treatment is available, we have adapted guidelines originally produced by the British Paediatric Association for unorthodox treatments.

The Committee is aware that children with learning disabilities are particularly vulnerable and that some treatment strategies have the potential to be applied abusively. We have made some recommendations to minimise this possibility.

Parents and staff who deal with children with learning disabilities and challenging behaviour made it clear to the Committee that they see a need to acquire new treatment skills. In addition to regular training to increase their competencies, they also want access to good quality supervision and support.

6.1.1 Developmental issues

A developmental understanding informs most of the treatment approaches mentioned in this chapter. The child's behaviour and its significance are viewed in a developmental context.

Children with learning disabilities need access to a range of developmental opportunities where they can acquire new skills. Teaching children new developmentally appropriate skills is desirable in itself and may reduce challenging behaviour. Children with severe learning disabilities are less likely than other children to interact spontaneously with their physical environment. They are more likely to need other people to encourage and structure this kind of exploration, which is part of normal child development. A child with poor play skills who habitually, for example, destroys toys will need assistance to use them more positively for interesting and developmentally valuable experiences. Skills teaching has the added bonus that it will involve the child interacting with another person. This may help them become more socially responsive and better able to communicate in acceptable ways.

Children with learning disabilities, like all children, have feelings and emotions and form relationships with other people. For any treatment intervention to succeed the child must feel reasonably safe and contained within a secure, reliable relationship. Anyone providing treatment, for their part, must respect and value the child and be ready to listen to and face the feelings that emerge. Consent to treatment is important for all interventions and requires parents and children to be given accurate, clear information to enable them to make informed choices.

The Committee took a child centred approach. We recognise that there will be occasions where the needs of the parent, the child and the services differ. There is a need for the child's needs and wishes to be specifically addressed. This may require the identification of an independent advocate for the child.

6.1.2 Evidence base

There were concerns in many of the responses received about the current lack of clear evidence for the efficacy of particular treatment approaches. Parents want to know whether treatment really works. Commissioners and purchasers are seeking evidence of 'value for money'. Both want rapid and effective achievement of clearly specified outcome measures.

A number of correspondents highlighted the difficulties in providing information of this quality for this group of children. Children with learning disabilities and severe challenging behaviour are a diverse group (see chapter 2). They differ in the causes of their disabilities and the causes of their challenging behaviour as well as in many other respects. They are also very vulnerable. Their problems are both very disabling and rare. There are therefore considerable ethical and methodological difficulties in conducting a randomised double blind controlled trial. The Committee was not aware of any research based on intention to treat. We simply do not know how many children drop out of treatment programmes especially at an early stage.

The evidence we do have is mainly, therefore, based on single case experiments, group studies and meta-analyses of such experiments, a few controlled trials on rather heterogeneous groups of children and single case reports. The Committee also used evidence from other groups, particularly children without learning disabilities and adults with learning disabilities and severe challenging behaviour.

The evidence that behavioural treatments reduce the frequency and severity of challenging behaviour is compelling. There is some evidence that medication is effective for specific indications. Other treatments may well work for individual children, but there is less scientific evidence regarding their efficacy. In practice treatment tends to be given as part of a package consisting of several individual treatments, education and family support. Research is often directed at particular components of the packages. Much less is known about how such packages work.

6.1.3 Outcomes

The main aim of treatment, as defined above, is to reduce the frequency, duration or intensity of the challenging behaviour itself. Treatment may also result in a number of other outcomes which improve the child's quality of life and may reduce the extent to which a particular behaviour is seen as 'challenging', even when the behaviour is unaltered. These desirable outcomes can, in principle, be measured and used to evaluate treatment.

Desirable outcomes of treatment

- reduction in frequency
  - duration
  - intensity of challenging behaviour
- acquisition of new skills by the child
- integration/reintegration of child into
  - education
  - leisure activities
  - family life
- return child to more local facilities
  - prevent inappropriate use of distant facilities
- change way behaviour is viewed
  - in the family
  - at school
  - by wider community
- improve competency of parents
  - teachers
  - other service staff
- reduction in use of restraint
  - sedation

6.1.4 Further research

The Committee concluded that there was an urgent need for further research in this area. In particular funding bodies should be looking to commission intervention studies in community settings with agreed outcome criteria. They should also encourage researchers to develop methodologies to identify criteria for deciding which treatment(s) to use with which child and the effectiveness of packages of treatment.

6.1.5 Staff training supervision and support

Challenging behaviour by definition poses a challenge to services. Staff may feel upset, angry, disgusted or overwhelmed by aspects of a child's behaviour. Staff, therefore, need both up to date training in the specific competencies that will enable them to help the child and good support and supervision. This must also be available to parents when they are acting as therapists. The Committee was told of gaps and deficits in the training of both professional and unqualified staff.

The Committee believes that the DoH and the DfEE should jointly establish nationally agreed and enforceable standards for the training and qualifications of staff working in health, social care, education and other services for children with severe challenging behaviour.

6.1.6 The Context for Treatment

The Committee was aware of a number of other issues which acted as a backdrop to our discussions:

- Local services vary enormously in the way they are organised, the way they handle referrals, the treatments that are available and the level and type of support offered.
- There is considerable professional debate about optimum models for identifying, assessing, treating and reviewing challenging behaviour.
- Treatment should be based on evidence that it works both in general and for the particular child.
- Treatment must therefore be regularly reviewed.
- There is uncertainty about legally permissible treatments with the consequent danger of some children receiving no treatment at all.

In making recommendations, the Committee was continually aware of its commitment to child-centred services. These should be as inclusive as possible while being able to offer the very specialist help which these children required, sometimes on a continuing or very long-term basis.

The Committee believes that whatever treatment is provided, it should be flexible, tailored to the needs of the individual child, regularly reviewed, responsive to parental views and as near to the child's home as possible.

6.2 Timing of treatment

6.2.1 Early intervention

The Committee heard from many respondents that it was desirable to start treatment as early as possible, to prevent behaviour patterns becoming more fixed and harder to change over time. Indeed, many of those who gave evidence and the Committee itself, hoped that intervention before the child first showed behaviour problems, might prevent the development of challenging behaviour altogether. The Committee, therefore, commissioned a literature review on this subject. We concluded that there is evidence to show that early intervention can help young children with learning disabilities develop new skills. However, there is as yet little evidence that such programmes can prevent some children with a learning disability developing challenging behaviour. There are some recent reports that suggest that skill building may itself prevent challenging behaviour in some children (Emerson 1996). Early intervention was greatly appreciated by parents and may have helped them cope better later. Since it would obviously be better to devise preventative interventions than only to intervene after behaviour was perceived to be challenging, the Committee agreed that there was an urgent need for outcome based research in the area of interventions with very young children with a learning disability and their families. Although we believe there is a strong theoretical case for early interventions, which can prevent or ameliorate challenging behaviours in very young children with learning disabilities, there is a lack of information about the kind of services which might best help these children and their families.

We urge grant awarding bodies to commission further research on:

- early intervention and early detection of challenging behaviour;
- the short and longer-term effectiveness of early behavioural and other interventions, at the level of the individual child;
- the conditions under which such interventions are undertaken;
- the factors which may affect whether or not family and community services persist with interventions;
- the development of training strategies for parents and providers of pre-school services in order to contribute to the identification of challenging behaviour and the effective implementation of behavioural or other interventions.

6.2.2 Early intervention for established challenging behaviour

The Committee heard that once behaviour that is seen to be challenging develops, an intervention should be made as soon as possible. The Committee identified a number of reasons for this:

- Because young children are rarely threatening and their behaviour may be less stigmatising, they are more likely to be successfully integrated into enriching social and educational environments.
- Parents and teachers may find it easier to remove smaller children from situations when necessary, something more difficult when they are older and stronger.
- The longer a particular behaviour has been allowed to go on the more likely it is to have been reinforced in many situations. It will come to serve many functions for the child and become harder to change.
- Behaviour that is easily tolerated in a young child, eg stripping, throwing things, may be very challenging indeed in a large adolescent.
- Challenging behaviour is often painful and distressing for the child and for this reason alone, early intervention is not only justifiable, but desirable.

The Committee concluded that that the three statutory authorities, education, health and social services, must work together. All Children's Services Plans should contain specific proposals for multi- agency initiatives to ensure:

- that all families have early access to practical and appropriate support and advice which can help them manage any emerging or actual behaviour difficulties;
- that all young children with learning disabilities who show signs of behavioural difficulties should have a full, multi-agency assessment at the earliest opportunity;
- following assessment, children who require specialist support should be referred to the appropriate services without delay;
- that the three authorities develop shared strategic approaches and agreed criteria for the referral of young children to specialist tertiary services or centres.

The Committee believes that LEAs should ensure that nursery schools and classes and other providers of pre-school provision have access to appropriate advice and support from their local educational psychology service to support young children with challenging behaviour. This should include addressing the training and support needs of pre-school teaching and non-teaching staff.

6.3 Multi-disciplinary, multi-agency assessment

Most respondents favoured a multi-agency, multi-disciplinary approach. Treatment should be initiated following thorough assessment. However, the Committee heard of many cases where a child had been repeatedly assessed, but no treatment was forthcoming. Our overwhelming impression was of gaps and holes in services rather than duplication of effort. For example, about 20 per cent of posts in child psychology and at least 30 per cent of posts in psychology of learning disability are vacant. Only 23 per cent of trainees in mental handicap psychiatry (now psychiatry of learning disability) felt that their training was adequate to offer a service to children and only 13 per cent of trainees in child psychiatry felt adequately prepared to offer a service to children with severe learning disabilities. In Harris and Upton's study, though teachers described many pupils in schools for children with severe learning disability as showing challenging behaviour, few teachers expected that there would be help from any agency outside the school.

Most worryingly parents often gained little help. Qureshi's (1993) work on young adults with challenging behaviour showed that 26 per cent of parents felt they had had no advice from professionals and a further 61 per cent had had no advice that they found helpful. Only 13 per cent of parents felt they had received useful advice from any professional about their child's challenging behaviour.

The lack of coordination between treatment services was also seen as a problem by parents and professionals. Many parents responding to the Committee reported on the negative impact of multiple sources of advice, with some parents seeing as many as 20 different professionals within a year. Some contributors felt strongly that treatment should be coordinated by a particular service: the child development centre, the child mental health services, the learning disability services or the school; or under the leadership of a particular professional, clinical psychologist (child or learning disability), consultant psychiatrist (child or learning disability), or community paediatrician. No clear consensus emerged about the optimum model for an effective service. There was general agreement that improved collaboration and coordination between and within all three statutory services was essential.

The Committee recognised that in different parts of the country health services for this group of children had developed in different ways. Health services for children with learning disabilities and challenging behaviour may be led from child and adolescent mental health services, learning disability services or child development centres. Wherever health services are based, there must be regular liaison with education and social services. All three services must ensure that parents, schools and relevant professionals are aware of their existence and that access is straightforward.

The Committee suggests that health service commissioners look critically at existing services and identify the lead health provider. They should then build on the strengths of existing services, seeking to incorporate relevant expertise from other services. There should also be a single, easily accessible entry point to these services.

6.4 Where is treatment provided?

As we have argued elsewhere in the report, a tiered approach to services is necessary. Most treatment should be home or school based. Where highly specialist investigation or treatment is needed children with learning disabilities and challenging behaviour must have equality of access. This will include access to neuro-psychiatric services. (See also chapters 2 and 8)

6.5 Families

The great majority of children with learning disabilities and challenging behaviour live with their families. Parents, brothers and sisters often spend more hours with the child than anyone else. They know the child well and develop strong views about the child's needs as well as their own. As they told the Committee, they want recognition, support, information and to be involved in decision making.

6.5.1 Parents as therapists

The past decade has seen major changes and developments with parental involvement both in the assessment and in a range of treatment and interventions to help their children. The Committee was given a number of examples of parents themselves providing the 'hands on treatment', sometimes with professional support and supervision, but sometimes without such guidance. They defined 'treatment' broadly as engaging in activities which were over and above the usual responsibilities and tasks of parenthood. A number of recent evaluations of parent involvement in early intervention programmes – in particular Portage – have demonstrated the effectiveness of parents as therapists (Sylvan, 1993; Cameron, 1992). Parental involvement facilitates active working partnerships. Parents are, in any event, likely to have the best overall knowledge of their child and the success (or otherwise) of various interventions in the context of the child's home.

The Code of Practice and the 1996 Education Act give parents greatly enhanced opportunities (and responsibilities) to share in assessment and planning. Some very positive parent advice and befriending schemes also demonstrate the effectiveness of the voluntary sector, in providing peer support and advice for potentially isolated or vulnerable families. Nonetheless an increasing number of parents are highlighting their aspirations to be 'parents first'.

'Our lives are utterly abnormal, because of the pressure of compliance with different professionals' expectations. Of course we do comply. We don't want to lose a service! But couldn't professionals work as a team to help all of us prioritise what services we are going to use and which treatment we will all try? Sometimes I feel we live in a programme, not a home. If you were a child, would you want to come home to a programme?' (A parent)

Our evidence reinforced the view that parents want partnership. They want an equal, respected and valued working relationship and they wish to be part of any treatment or therapy approach. They need to be involved on equal terms, ie given opportunities for training, able to negotiate how, when and where they work and to have explanations not instructions. Some parents noted that treatment approaches might imply very different life-styles to their own, eg carpets to provide soundproofing, separate bedrooms, a parent at home all day, no other siblings with competing demands, a car and a telephone.

The Committee believes that home based treatments must be sensitive to the circumstances of the individual family and their social/cultural beliefs. Parents should be offered adequate explanations, training and continuing support in any intervention they are expected to carry out.

6.5.2 Family support and counselling

Different forms of parental counselling or family work were mentioned many times in evidence and considerable importance attributed to these kinds of interventions. Again there is or should be a tiered approach. Several parents mentioned support from other parents. Others had found health visitors or community nurses very helpful. Most of the evidence described support and counselling which helped the families cope with challenging behaviour. There was much less evidence about helping families to address possible family issues which might be contributing to the challenging behaviour. It is important that services do not contribute to parents feeling 'blamed' for their child's challenging behaviour.

Family therapy as such is used in some services for some families. The therapy focuses on the relationships between family members. Therapy may be used to help the family deal with the impact of the child's disabilities. In some families, however, other issues such as employment or marital relationships will turn out to be more relevant (eg Vetere, 1993).

6.5.3 Family involvement in treatment decisions

Parents told the Committee that they wanted to be involved in decisions about their child's treatment. Service providers broadly welcomed this. The legal position on consent is covered elsewhere (see chapter 7). Parents particularly welcomed honest information from service providers. Few treatments for challenging behaviour will be effective immediately and in many instances a number of different interventions will need to be tried, evaluated and pursued or rejected. Some parents told us that they found it very difficult and demoralising to persist with treatments that did not appear to work. They felt inadequate and upset at disappointing the professionals. One parent said that it would be much better to be honest.

'Sometimes we may have a particular priority for a behaviour which is not yours - ask us. Enabling a child to travel on the bus or to give parents some sleep may be the key to a lot more participation and a much more supportive family! Equally all of us feel very strongly about prioritising intervention for behaviours which might exclude our children from school. It is not just parents who can feel isolated. Teachers and other professionals can too – I have a dual rôle as teacher and parent and I often feel isolated and marginalised in both.'

Service providers have a responsibility to make information available to parents and children, so that they can make informed decisions about treatment.

6.6 Choice of treatment(s)

Some services use a single treatment model, while others use a combination of different approaches. Evidence received by the Committee indicated that service providers generally support an eclectic approach that can offer a coherent package individually tailored to the needs of the child and family and rigorously monitored and reviewed. Any treatment should be based on one or more hypotheses about the causes and functions of the behaviour. Treatment can then be directed at testing out these possible explanations.

Employing an eclectic approach and making a range of treatments available has advantages as well as drawbacks.

On the one hand:

▶ parents and children can exercise choice about treatment options;
▶ individual children can respond differently to the same treatment approach and what suits one child may well not be right for another;
▶ even where a child is thought likely to benefit from a particular form of treatment, there may be complex reasons for the behaviour which require more than one type of intervention.

On the other hand:

▶ staff using a range of treatments may have too little experience of using one approach to develop real proficiency in using it;
▶ when one approach appears not to be working, it may be tempting to move on to another treatment model rather than modifying the first strategy to see if it can be made more effective;

▶ there can be a tendency to seize on new treatments which may be ineffective or even harmful.

The Committee believes it is highly unlikely that a single type of treatment is suitable for all children with learning disabilities and challenging behaviour. The Committee supports the following recommendations, produced in the USA at the National Institutes of Health Consensus Development Conference on Treatment of Destructive Behaviours in Persons with Developmental Disabilities, held in 1989:

▶ Most successful treatments are likely to involve multiple elements of therapy (behavioural and psychopharmacologic), environment change and education.

▶ Treatment methods may require techniques for enhancing desired behaviours, for producing changes in social, physical and educational environments and for reducing or eliminating destructive behaviours.

▶ Treatments should be based on an analysis of medical and psychiatric conditions, environmental situations, consequences and skill deficits. In the application of any of these treatments, an essential step involves a functional analysis of existing behaviour patterns.

▶ Behaviour reduction procedures should be selected for their rapid effectiveness, only if the exigencies of the clinical situation require such restrictive interventions and only after appropriate review. These interventions should only be used in the context of a comprehensive treatment package (NIH, 1990)

Services should choose a particular treatment option on the basis of existing evidence about its efficacy. While it is important to offer choice to children and their parents, this should not mean that treatments of proven efficacy are unavailable, because scarce human or financial resources have been directed to more innovative treatment whose effectiveness is unknown.

The Committee was repeatedly told that it is important for services offering treatment in homes and schools to be sensitive to the social and cultural context and to the competing demands on parents and teachers.

The various behaviourally based approaches have been more systematically evaluated than any other methods of treatment, not least because detailed recording of behaviour is an integral part of these approaches, thus offering a readily available and rich source of data. The studies are, for the most part, single case studies or relatively small samples. There are very few studies that include other clinical information that might influence treatment outcome (such as family circumstances, psychiatric disorders). Relatively few studies describe work undertaken in the child's own home or class-room. It is not known how many of the schools or families offered behavioural intervention accept it and how many either refuse or fail to implement behavioural advice.

Although evidence about the relative efficacy of different treatments can be an important factor in decision-making about treatment options, choice of treatment, the Committee heard, was sometimes also partly determined by a service's philosophical objections to particular methods or approaches and a few went so far as to ban a particular treatment completely. Where this occurred it seems to have been either because the organisation was very conscious of the potential for abuse with a particular treatment, or that they were wary of applying a single treatment to all children, without first addressing the issue of why the particular child behaved in that way in a particular time and place.

While the Committee shared these concerns, we did not feel that services should place a total ban on effective techniques (eg behaviour modification and drugs). Rather they should ensure that monitoring was in place and that abuse could be prevented.

The Committee concluded that there must be inter-agency monitoring of children's behaviour and development and accurate recordings of behaviour. The effectiveness, or otherwise, of particular interventions should be shared with all concerned with the child and used to evaluate the effectiveness of different forms of treatment.

The Committee was concerned that the use of any control, restraint or potentially controversial treatment should be carefully reviewed and only used in the context of a wider diagnosis, assessment and care plan for the particular child. Accurate and effective assessment and diagnosis should be the cornerstone of any challenging behaviour policy.

Concern was also expressed about whether certain treatments might be considered abusive. Several recent cases which have received media attention have demonstrated the importance of ensuring that all services working with children with challenging behaviour give careful consideration to ethical as well as legal issues when contemplating interventions involving restraint or aversion. (Harris J. 1996)

We recommend that treatment should always be based on a clear analysis of the causes of the behaviour and that full consideration of possible explanations should precede any treatment. Assessment should lead on to a decision about active treatment and should not be seen as an end in itself.

In deciding whether a particular treatment should be used for a particular child the Committee suggests the following considerations are taken into account. They are based on guidelines originally issued by the British Paediatric Association for unorthodox treatments. The Committee added to them so that they can be used more generally.

- The scientific plausibility of the programme proposed;
- the evidence for its effectiveness;
- the methods to be used in measuring and evaluating outcome;
- the extent to which parents may benefit from the opportunity to try the method they prefer;
- the possible adverse effects of the programme on the child or family;
- the impact of treatment, including time costs to child and family;
- the extent to which the parents and child are informed of the possible benefits and risks of the treatment;
- the right of parents (and children) to choose;
- the difference in potential benefit between programmes;
- where the proposed treatment is to be funded by statutory services, whether the magnitude of the difference can justify the difference in costs.

(Adapted from BPA, 1994)

6.7 Treatment approaches

6.7.1 Behavioural approaches

Behavioural approaches are based on the principles of learning theory, but in fact may be effective even when the causes of a particular behaviour is a biochemical brain abnormality (eg Lesch-Nyhan syndrome).

Behavioural approaches seek:

▶ to eliminate or minimise the specific triggers for problem behaviours;
▶ present or emphasise triggers that increase the likelihood of more appropriate behaviours;
▶ present or emphasise triggers that inhibit the occurrence of problem behaviours;
▶ minimise the intensity and duration of these behaviours once they have started.

A behavioural approach is also used to understand the functions of a behaviour, that is the settings, triggers and consequences that make a particular behaviour more likely to occur in future. This functional behavioural analysis underpins modern behavioural treatments. There is no longer any place for behavioural treatments based on the form of the behaviour eg aggression, self injury, that do not take account of function. One child may injure himself when he is asked to join in a classroom activity, another may be more likely to hurt herself when she is left alone. Treatment must be based on an understanding of the functions of particular behaviour for the particular child. Challenging behaviour may in fact be an adaptive means to an end for a child who has not acquired more socially and developmentally appropriate ways of achieving this. As noted in Chapter 2, children with learning disabilities may not have learned appropriate behaviours because of their impairments, lack of social responsiveness and communication difficulties.

Functional behavioural analysis and a behavioural approach may be used to manipulate the environment or to identify new skills a child needs, as well as providing a way of working directly on the challenging behaviour.

Carr (1994) has described the assumptions that underlie positive behavioural support:

- challenging behaviour usually serves a purpose for the person who displays it;
- prior to intervention, functional assessment should be used to try to identify the purpose of challenging behaviour;
- the goal of education is to educate and to introduce new skills, not simply to reduce challenging behaviour;
- intervention involves changing social systems, such as schools or the ways families interact, rather than just changing the person with challenging behaviour (as such intervention is best carried out in the places in which people normally live, learn and work);
- the ultimate goal of intervention is to improve people's quality of life or lifestyle, not just to reduce challenging behaviour.

Setting for behavioural treatments

Although functional analyses of behaviour may be carried out in a clinic or other 'service' setting, they are increasingly being modified for use in the child's natural settings such as home or school, since children may behave quite differently in different settings. Behaviour learned in a clinic may not generalise to other settings. It is therefore preferable to carry out the behavioural interventions at home or school for maximum potential benefit. The rôle of the professional will then be to advise and support those in daily contact with the child to record and respond to particular behaviours consistently. This places a considerable burden on families and school staff but it is necessary if treatment is to succeed.

Consistent responses from other people are important if the child is to benefit from the treatment. This implies exceptionally good communication between all those involved with the child. For some children this will need to involve siblings, dinner ladies and bus drivers as well as parents, teachers and care staff. It also assumes that family members, teachers and other key figures are willing and able to work in this way.

For a very small number of children there may need to be a degree of consistency across the twenty-four hours that can only be achieved in an extremely specialist residential school.

Long-term interventions

Treatment to help a child through a particular problem, especially if the child learns new ways of achieving the same result through teaching or development, is often extremely effective. On the other hand, achieving and sustaining behavioural change can be difficult. Behavioural approaches may need to be used consistently for many years. One-off treatment episodes are unlikely to produce lasting positive effects where behaviour is severely challenging. The Committee received evidence that for some people with learning disabilities, severe challenging behaviour will persist into adulthood, even where a person has had high quality behavioural interventions during childhood. This implies that all those carrying out behavioural interventions will need continuing access to support and supervision.

Environmental manipulation

Functional analysis may suggest changes to a child's environment that would reduce the likelihood of a particular behaviour occurring or lessen the risks to the child if it does. These may be quite minor changes, such as altering where a child sits in a class room or reducing the level of noise. For children with autism the environment may need to be free from distractions and very predictable.

Children may also need environmental alteration for their own protection. For example, parents of young children often fit locks to cupboards and remove sharp objects.

The Committee visited two specialist units where extensive environmental manipulation is used. Toughened window panes, televisions with perspex screens and pictures screwed to the wall obviously make sense when children throw objects around. Similarly, providing furniture without sharp edges may be necessary if children are prone to self-injury. However, such measures could easily become unnecessarily restrictive.

The Committee believes that a small number of children with severe learning disabilities and severe challenging behaviour are at risk of serious injury to themselves or others unless they live in a physical environment that would be considered abnormal. This should be seen as a legitimate part of treatment, but the aim should always be for children to have access to as normal an environment as is consistent with their own and others' safety.

The Committee believes that that where adaptations to a child's physical environment and daily living arrangements are considered necessary, both the risks posed and the effectiveness of any treatment of this kind must be regularly reviewed to avoid unnecessary restriction.

Aversive treatments

The Committee was particularly concerned that one class of behavioural treatment had considerable potential for abuse. Aversive treatments are defined as any behavioural treatment that makes use of an aversive stimulus that the individual consistently avoids or escapes.(Johnston 1988). The Committee was particularly concerned about those aversive treatments which involve:

- the infliction of physical pain;

and/or

- produce effects that require medical attention;

and/or

- are judged to be outside the norms for how people in society should treat one another.

(Horner, 1990; Murphy, 1993)

The Committee therefore believes that:

- clear guidelines should exist to prevent the use of aversive treatments as defined by Horner and Murphy, save in exceptional circumstances;
- aversive treatments should be used very cautiously, if at all, and only on the basis of clear assessment and agreed outcome criteria;
- the consent of the parents and of the child, if he/she has the capacity, must be obtained before aversive treatment can be used;
- the decision to embark on such a treatment programme should only be made by a multi-disciplinary meeting of senior clinicians following multi-disciplinary assessment;
- aversive treatments should only be contemplated where they are thought to be the least detrimental alternative;
- aversive treatments should never be instigated by a single member of staff acting on their own or by junior staff.

Respondents also pointed out that it could be difficult to know how to rate events which occur outside any planned treatment interventions (eg shouting at a child).

Communication-based approaches

As noted in Chapters 2 and 4, there is considerable support for the view that children with communication difficulties may use challenging behaviour to convey their feelings, wants and needs to others (eg by screaming or hitting someone). Even children with speech may have difficulty making themselves understood, perhaps using inappropriate language. Behavioural approaches can be used to teach communication skills. Several studies have demonstrated that self-injury or aggression can be reduced by teaching individuals to use signs or simple phrase as alternative and more appropriate means of communication. These can be used to ask for help, for example, or to request a brief break from a task.

Challenging behaviour can however develop in a child who has apparently good communication skills.

With varying levels of support from empirical evidence, all techniques which seek to enhance social responsiveness as a basis for establishing relationships claim success. Given the potential importance of relationships in averting the development of challenging behaviour, these approaches deserve further rigorous study.

6.7.2 Drug treatment

There seemed a consensus that drugs could sometimes be useful but that there was a risk that they could be abused and that drug administration caused very practical difficulties across services. The evidence for the effectiveness of particular drugs often comes by analogy with other groups of people: children without learning disabilities, adults, or from single case studies. There is very little research on the effectiveness of medication specifically in children with learning disabilities.

Drugs may be used to control behaviour or to treat a specific disorder. There is good

Einfeld's Checklist on the Prescription of Psychotropic Medication

- The decision to prescribe psychotropic medication should follow a comprehensive assessment of the individual's emotional and behavioural disturbance.
- Proper consideration should be given to the issue of informed consent.
- Treatment with psychotropic drugs needs to be an integrated part of other concurrent treatments.
- Integrating psychotropic medication with other treatment modalities requires good inter-disciplinary communication.
- The precise symptoms for which the psychotropic medication is being prescribed should be stated.
- There should be some rationale to suggest that the drugs to be prescribed are likely to be useful for the target symptoms.
- One needs to establish some method for reliably and validly documenting changes in the target symptoms during the course of treatment.
- This record should demonstrate that target symptoms have had a positive response to the medication before the drug is continued.
- When the initially prescribed dose has failed to produce improvements, increases in dosage should not continue beyond a predetermined maximum level.
- When target symptoms have been reduced or absent for a reasonable period then an attempt should be made to reduce the dose being administered.
- When a psychotropic medication is withdrawn, a proper withdrawal regime should be designed.
- Because of the presence of organic brain dysfunction, the response to psychotropic drugs is often relatively idiosyncratic.
- Because of the often idiosyncratic response to psychotropics, their administration should be regarded to some extent as a therapeutic trial.
- As with any other individual, general principles of pharmacotherapy need to be observed including issues of compliance, drug absorption and excretion, drug interactions and side effects.

NB. Specifying and monitoring a target behaviour is not always easy and requires the same rigor as any other behavioural assessment, it depends on the understanding and goodwill of parents and teachers to carry it out.

(Einfeld, 1990)

---

evidence that specific drugs can be useful in treating epilepsy and specific psychiatric disorders, such as depression and attention deficit disorder. There is also increasing interest in basing drug treatments on an understanding of the functions of the behaviour, for example, in using opiate blocking drugs to treat self injury.

The Committee, perhaps surprisingly, heard some arguments for the use of drugs simply to control behaviour. The arguments were often based on the needs of the rest of the family. There may be a need for this kind of treatment, but it often reflects the non-availability of other services.(Hubert, 1992; Hogg, 1992). The Committee believes that drugs should only be used in this way when they are the least detrimental alternative and that other solutions should be actively pursued.

Drug treatment of specific conditions can be very effective (eg Sturmey, 1995; Campbell, 1995) and should be available to children with learning disabilities and challenging behaviour after appropriate multi-disciplinary assessment. Because of underlying brain damage each treatment is, to some extent, a therapeutic trial. There is also evidence that some children remain on medication, unreviewed for many years, which is potentially dangerous and quite unacceptable.

The Committee therefore believes that:

▶ Sedation should only be prescribed for children with learning disabilities and challenging behaviour as part of a more comprehensive treatment programme; in an emergency until a comprehensive assessment and treatment package can be set up; or for specific medical and dental procedures (eg CT scanning).

▶ Considerable caution should be exercised by paediatricians and general practitioners (GPs) in prescribing and monitoring psychotropic medication for children with learning disabilities and challenging behaviour. Specialist psychiatric advice should be sought if such treatment is considered (BPA, 1994). Clear guidelines must be drawn up about which doctor is responsible for writing prescriptions and monitoring drug effects (wanted and unwanted).

▶ This implies that all children with learning disabilities and challenging behaviour, including those in boarding schools, should have access to psychiatric help.

▶ All service providers must be trained, supported and supervised so that they can continue any drug that is being provided by parents at home.

▶ Consent issues must be properly addressed whenever drugs are prescribed.

▶ It is essential that prescribed medication is regularly reviewed and its effects on behaviour systematically recorded.

Checklists, such as that prepared by Einfeld or the adapted version in 'Legal Issues arising from the Care, Control and Safety of Children with Learning Disabilities who also Present Severe Challenging Behaviour' (Lyon, C, 1994) may be helpful in outlining responsible prescribing.

6.7.3 Psychotherapeutic treatments

The Committee heard of cognitive and psychodynamic psychotherapies being used with children with learning disabilities and challenging behaviours. Although these treatments are generally more difficult to evaluate than behavioural programmes, we know that psychotherapy is used and highly valued by some families and children.

In some services psychotherapeutic treatment is offered as part of a treatment package, alongside other approaches. This requires effective collaboration between all the professionals involved and may be unfamiliar to psychotherapists, who have not worked with children with learning disabilities and challenging behaviour before.

Individual and group psychotherapies are being used with children with learning disabilities and challenging behaviour. The Committee was not aware of any studies that showed an effect on challenging behaviour for groups of children, though Birchard, Sinason and Usiskin (1996) have demonstrated an encouraging improvement in other areas of function.

Psychodynamic psychotherapy

'Psychodynamic psychotherapy, which may be individual, group or family based, is described as 'a form of treatment in which the relationship between the child and the therapist is central to the treatment process. Psychotherapists use this relationship to try to enable the child to change his/her behaviour by understanding it. With the exception of children with certain syndromes (eg Lesch-Nyhan and Prader-Willi), psychotherapists would broadly understand challenging behaviour as an expression of unmanageable anxiety and confusion.' (Wilson, 1997).

There are case reports that suggest psychodynamic psychotherapy may be helpful in reducing the extent of challenging behaviour in children with learning disabilities. Though children with learning disabilities have traditionally been regarded as unsuitable for this kind of psychotherapy because of their intellectual impairment and/or limited verbal capacity, there is some clinical evidence that it can be useful. Harris, for example, states that

'psychotherapeutic interventions are most effective in the treatment of emotional and behavioural disturbance in individuals who have had traumatic psychosocial experiences. Individual psychotherapy may consist of a variety of specific approaches and techniques, depending on the ability and intellect of the child and the skills of the therapist. Cognitive techniques may be used with some children and/or at different points in the treatment'.

Psychotherapy research is more difficult to carry out than behavioural research. Nonetheless the Committee believes that psychotherapy must be evaluated to see whether it is effective, both for the particular child and more generally. Treatment of this kind should be regularly monitored against agreed outcome measures, not least because it is extremely time consuming for the child and parent as well as the therapists. Further rigorous research is needed in this area.

6.7.4 Creative therapies

The Committee received a number of submissions about music therapy, art therapy and drama therapy. Although not necessarily used specifically to 'treat' challenging behaviour, respondents pointed out how these approaches could help a child establish a relationship with an adult. Very withdrawn children may be more engaged during a music therapy session, for example. Even where the therapy may not lead to any particular improvement in behaviour, it can sometimes contribute to a better quality of life.

6.8 Alternative or complementary treatments

In addition to the range of treatment approaches described above, the Committee was aware that some parents may consider one of the growing number of 'alternative' and less orthodox treatments. Some treatments, such as aromatherapy massage, acupuncture and cranial osteopathy are beginning to be used quite widely as complementary treatments to more orthodox interventions and are being systematically evaluated. Others could be described as more 'fringe treatments'. Parents whose child has severe challenging behaviour may be willing to try anything, particularly if previous interventions have failed to modify difficult behaviour. It may also enable parents to feel that they are taking some responsibility for their child's welfare rather than allowing professionals to 'take over'.

This is understandable. But the Committee is concerned that parents should not expose their child to potential abuse (recognising, of course, that abuse can also occur with orthodox treatments). Children with challenging behaviour should never be exposed to treatments which place them at risk of physical or psychological harm.

Good parent-professional relationships should enable parents to feel comfortable enough to discuss with the professionals treating their child any alternative approaches they may be considering. The possible pros and cons can then be discussed in an open and honest way so that, hopefully, a decision is reached which is in the best interests of the child.

We propose that the use of any alternative treatment should be considered within the framework of the adapted British Paediatric Association guidelines described earlier.

Recommendations

▶ Service commissioners and providers should ensure that whatever treatment is provided, it should be flexible and tailored to the needs of the individual child.

▶ Service providers must ensure that parents are informed and consulted in treatment decisions.

▶ The three statutory authorities, education, health and social services, must work together to ensure that treatment packages are based on comprehensive assessment and diagnosis.

▶ Service commissioners should ensure that, wherever possible, treatment should be home- and/or school-based and within the child's own community.

▶ Service providers must ensure that parents are consulted in treatment decisions.

▶ Health service commissioners should ensure that all children and families have access to assessment and treatment services with multi-disciplinary staffing including community nursing, clinical psychology, paediatric and psychiatric expertise.

▶ Service providers must review all treatments together with objective evidence of their effectiveness in the particular child. Because treatment for children with challenging behaviour and learning disabilities often needs to be long-term, the Committee recommends that all services develop clear policies for the maintenance and review of all treatment interventions.

▶ Service providers, purchasers, parents and children should be made aware that for some children very long-term interventions may be needed to prevent the child's behaviour challenging services at a later stage.

▶ Health service commissioners should look critically at existing services and identify the lead health provider. They should then build on the strengths of existing services, seeking to incorporate relevant expertise from other services.

▶ Health services commissioners should identify a single, easily accessible, entry point to these services.

- Providers must ensure that they train, support and supervise all those carrying out treatment interventions, including parents and unqualified staff.
- Service providers must make information available to parents and children to help them make informed decisions about treatment.
- Commissioners and service providers should develop guidelines about the use of restraint, environmental manipulation, aversive treatment medication and other interventions that have the potential to be used abusively.
- Health service commissioners should ensure that children with learning disabilities and severe challenging behaviour have equality of access to specialist health services. This would include in-patient neuro-psychiatric services for assessment and establishment of treatment programmes for the small number of children with severe challenging behaviour and learning disabilities requiring this kind of provision.
- Research funding bodies should be looking to commission intervention studies, in community settings with agreed outcome criteria. They should also encourage researchers to develop methodologies to identify criteria for deciding which treatment(s) to use with which child and the effectiveness of packages of treatment.
- All children should have access to behavioural treatments based on a functional behavioural analysis and to medication. We further recommend that in the interests of increasing the choices available to children and parents, a range of other treatments is available including creative therapies and psychotherapy. Parents and children should be made aware that, at present, evidence on effectiveness is strongest for behavioural treatments and medication.
- Home based treatments should always be sensitive to the circumstances of the individual family and their social/cultural beliefs.

References

Aman MG (1993) Efficacy of psychotropic drugs for reducing self-injurious behaviour in the developmental disabilities (review). Annals of Clinical Psychiatry 5 (3): 171-188.

Baumeister AA Todd ME and Sevin JA (1993) Efficacy and specificity of pharmacological therapies for behavioural disorders in persons with mental retardation (review). Clinical Neuropharmacology, 16 (4): 271-294.

Birchard S.H Sinason V and Usiskin J (1996) Measuring change in mentally retarded clients in long-term psychoanalytic psychotherapy. National Association for the Dually Diagnosed 13: 6-11.

McKay I and Hall D et al. (1994) Services for children and adolescents with learning disability (mental handicap). London, British Paediatric Association.

Campbell M and Cueva JE (1995) Psychopharmacology in child and adolescent psychiatry: a review of the past seven years Part I (Review). Journal of the American Academy of Child and Adolescent Psychiatry 34 (9): 1124-1132.

Carr Edward G Levin L McConnachie G Carlson J I Kemp D C and Smith C E (1994) Communication-based intervention for problem behaviour: A user's guide for producing positive change. Baltimore MD Paul H. Brookes Publishing Co.

Einfeld S L (1990) Guidelines for the use of psychotropic medication in individuals with developmental disabilities. Australian & New Zealand Journal of Developmental Disabilities 16: 71-73.

Emerson E (1996) Early intervention autism and challenging behaviour. Tizard Learning Disability Review 1: 36-38.

Emerson E (1995) Challenging Behaviour Analysis and Intervention in People with Learning Disabilities. Cambridge, Cambridge University Press.

Emerson E. (1993) Challenging Behaviours and severe learning disabilities recent developments in behavioural analysis and intervention. Behavioural and Cognitive Psychotherapy 21, 171-198.

Gardner W I and Graeber J L (1993) Treatment of severe behavioural disorders in persons with mental retardation: A multimodal behavioural treatment model. In Mental Health Aspects of Mental Retardation Progress in Assessment and Treatment. Ed. R J Fletcher and A Dosen 201-241, New York, Lexington Books.

Gillberg C (1991) The Treatment of Epilepsy in Autism. Journal of Autism and Developmental Disorders 21: 61-77.

Harris J (1996) Physical restraint procedures for managing challenging behaviours presented by mentally retarded adults and children. Research in Developmental Disabilities 17 (2): 99-134.

Harris J Cook M Upton G (1996) Pupils with Severe Learning Disabilities who present Challenging Behaviour: A Whole School Approach to Assessment and Intervention. Worcester BILD Publications.

Harris J C (1995) Developmental Neuropsychiatry Volume II, Assessment Diagnosis and Treatment of Developmental Disorders. Oxford, Oxford University Press.

Hogg J (1992) The administration of psychotropic and anticonvulsant drugs to children with profound intellectual disability and multiple impairments. Journal of Intellectual Disability Research 36: 473-488.

Howlin P (in press) Treatment of Autism. Journal of Child Psychology and Psychiatry Practitioners Review.

Hubert J (1992) Too Many Drugs Too Little Care – Parent's perceptions of the administration and side effects of drugs prescribed for young people with severe learning difficulties. Values into Action.

Lyon C and Ashcroft E (1994) Legal Issues Arising from the Care and Control of Children with Learning Disabilities who also present Severe Challenging Behaviour. London, The Mental Health Foundation.

Murphy G H (1993) The use of aversive stimuli in treatment the issue of consent. Journal of Intellectual Disability Research 37 (3): 211-219.

National Institute of Health (1990) Consensus Conference on Treatment of Destructive Behaviours in Persons with Developmental Disabilities. Washington DC, US Government Printing Office.

Oliver C (1995) Annotation: self injurious behaviour in children with learning disability: recent advances in assessment and intervention. Journal of Child Psychology and Psychiatry 30 (6): 909-927.

Reiss S and Rojahn J (1993) Joint occurrence of depression and aggression in children and adults with mental retardation. Journal of Intellectual Disability Research 37: 287-294.

Repp A C, Felce D and Barton L E (1988) Basing the treatment of stereotypic and self-injurious behaviours of hypothesis of their causes. Journal of Applied Behavior Analysis 21: 281-289.

Rutter M, Hersov L.A and Taylor E (1993) Child and Adolescent Psychiatry: Modern approaches (3rd ed). Oxford, Blackwell.

Schaal D W and Hackenberg T (1994) Toward a functional analysis of drug treatment for behaviour problems of people with developmental disabilities (Review). American Journal of Mental Retardation 99 (2): 123-140.

Scotti J R, Evans I M, Meyer L H and Walker P (1991) A meta-analysis of intervention research with problem behavior treatment validity and standards of practice. American Journal of Mental Retardation 96: 233-256.

Sovner R and Lowry M .A (1990) A behavioural methodology for diagnosing affective disorders in individuals with mental retardation. In: 'Treatment of Mental Illness and Behavioural Disorder in the Mentally Retarded'. Ed. A Dosen A Van Gennep et al: 401-411, Amsterdam, Logon Publications.

Steen P L and Zuriff G E (1977) The use of relaxation in the treatment of self-injurious behaviour. Journal of Behavioural Therapy & Experiential Psychiatry 8: 447-448.

Turk J (1996) Working with parents of children who have severe learning disabilities. Clinical Child Psychology and Psychiatry 1 (4): 583-598.

Vetere A (1993) Using family therapy in services for people with learning disability. In: Using Family Therapy in the 90's. Ed. J Carpenter and A Treacher: 111-130.

Waitman A and Conboy-Hill S (1992) Psychotherapy and Mental Handicap. London, Sage.

Wolff S (1991) Childhood autism its diagnosis nature and treatment. Archives of Disease in Childhood 66: 737-741.

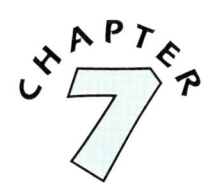

CHAPTER 7 The legal framework and other legal issues

The Legal Framework for Support Services

7.1 Introduction

The legal framework governing the provision of support services to families of children with learning disabilities who also present severe challenging behaviour is chiefly to be found in the Children Act (1989), which created a code of law concerning the upbringing of children. The Act aims to give all children (defined as anyone under the age of 18 years) the care, control and safety they require in their everyday lives. Although the Act contains a few provisions dealing with criminal procedure involving children, the primary focus of the legislation is more on domestic, welfare and social arrangements surrounding the care of children. There is, however, no specific mention in the Act of children with learning disabilities who also present severe challenging behaviour.

There are other provisions to support 'children in need' (section 17 Children Act (1989)) and their families and to protect all children in whatever environment they are being cared for, whether it is with their own family, within a foster or adoptive family, or by a childminder, in day care or in a children's home either private, voluntary or local authority (see Parts IV – XII Children Act (1989)). This duty to care for and protect children extends to children in hospitals, LEA residential establishments, in nursing homes for the mentally ill, as well as to children being accommodated in independent boarding schools (see sections 85 - 87 Children Act (1989)). All families, but especially those with children in need, should be able to look to the local authority support services for advice, assistance and support in coping. Through the provision of services, there should be no need for local authorities to intervene to protect the welfare of the child. The Act, however, does provide local authority social services with the means to remove the child from an environment in which they are believed to be suffering or at risk of suffering significant harm. For these purposes:

▶ 'harm' means the ill treatment or the impairment of helpful development;
▶ 'development' means physical, intellectual, emotional, social or behavioural development;
▶ 'health' means physical or mental health;
▶ 'ill treatment' includes sexual abuse and forms of ill treatment which are not physical (s.31(9) Children Act (1989)).

The Act further goes on to state that where the question whether harm suffered by a child is significant turns on the child's health or development, his health or development should be compared with that which could reasonably be expected of a similar child.

The key theme of the Children Act (1989) could therefore be said to be that children come first, that families matter, that parents should act responsibly, that there should be a mutually supportive partnership between parents of children in need and local authority agencies as well as health and education and that where children are at risk appropriate steps will be taken to protect them.

7.2 Part III Children Act (1989) and Part I Schedule 2

7.2.1 The definition of children in need and the duties towards such children

Part III of the Act (and specifically s.17(1)) imposes a general duty on every local authority to safeguard and promote the welfare of children in their area who are in need; and so far as is consistent with that duty, a further duty to promote the upbringing of such children by their family, by providing a range and level of services appropriate to those children's needs. S.17(10) of the Children Act (1989) defines a child in need as a child who is:

'Unlikely to achieve or maintain, or to have the opportunity of achieving or maintaining, a reasonable standard of health or development without the provision for him of services by the local authority under Part III of this Act.'

or

'his health or development is likely to be significantly impaired or further impaired without the provision for him of such services.'

or

'he is disabled.'

It is clear therefore that under the terms of this legislation children with learning disabilities and severely challenging behaviour fall entirely within this definition.

7.2.2 The expanded duty

The Act goes on to provide in s.17(2) that for the purposes of facilitating the discharge of their duties under s.17(1), every local authority has the specific duties and powers set out in Part 1 of Schedule 2. Indeed, the obligations laid upon local authorities, Part 1 of Schedule 2, are extremely detailed and do contain provisions specifically looking to the issues affecting children with disabilities. Thus, Schedule 2 Part 1 requires authorities to take reasonable steps to identify the extent to which there are children in need within their area and to publish information about services not only provided by them but also by voluntary organisations or other bodies. Local authorities are then required to open and maintain a register of disabled children and are also required to assess any child's needs for the purposes of this Act at the same time as other assessments are made under the Chronically Sick and Disabled Persons Act 1970; the Education Act (1996); the Disabled Persons (Services Consultation and Representation) Act 1986 and any other enactments.

As a number of reports (Audit Commission 1994; Children Act Reports 1992-1995) have pointed out, local authorities have struggled to publicise information widely about the services they provide and many of them have experienced difficulty over the maintenance of any register of disabled children.

As is evident throughout this report, there has also been a marked lack of coordination between the various agencies in terms of assessments of the needs of this particular group of children under the various pieces of legislation. Time and again evidence was presented to the Committee that education, social services and health appeared to be operating in total isolation from each other. It was clear that weak coordination across agencies in relation to definition of need under the different legislation, the different aims of the relevant services and their rôles in meeting the different kinds of vision all demand that there should be much greater coherence and shared planning in order to develop good quality local services which will meet the needs of these children in their families not only for the present but also for the future. Many groups and individual parents pointed to the fact that it appeared that a great many resources were being deployed by a range of different agencies, but not in the most efficient way.

Guidance issued by the DoH pursuant to the Children Act (1989) (DoH, 1991a) certainly recommended the establishment of joint planning committees to coordinate strategic planning and provision for children with disabilities, but it was quite apparent from evidence to the Committee that this had not been translated into such an approach across the country as a whole. There were isolated examples of good practice, but more remained to be done. Whilst the guidance stresses coordination and shared planning, it is clear that there should be some kind of joint case management system in which specialist (ie specially trained and expert) case managers could provide relatively long-term contact to families. This would require not only inter-agency cooperation but also a planned agreement to share resources which would ultimately result in their much more efficient deployment. This is particularly important in relation to this group of children.

7.2.3 The scope of local authority duties and responsibilities towards children in need

Part 1 of Schedule 2 also imposes upon local authorities a duty to ensure that services within this area are designed to minimise the effect on disabled children of their disabilities and give such children the opportunity to lead lives which are as normal as possible. Thus, under their general duties, local authorities must provide for children with learning disabilities and severe challenging behaviour. In allocating the services they are legally bound to provide, local authorities should give top priority to children with learning disabilities and severe challenging behaviour. Thus this group of children should be prioritised in terms of access to services which enable them to remain at home with their families, minimise the effect of their disabilities and enable them to lead lives which are as normal as possible.

It is quite clear from the evidence presented to the Committee and from some of the examples in this chapter that this has not necessarily been the experience of children with learning disabilities and severe challenging behaviour, even since the implementation of the Children Act (1989) in October 1991.

The clear message from the Children Act (1989) and in particular from Part III and Part 1 of Schedule 2, is that each child with learning disabilities and severe challenging behaviour should have their own specific package of care based on a coordinated and combined assessment but which is unique to their particular individual problems. Services which can be provided under the various pieces of legislation in the health, education and social welfare field may thus include:

▶ Portage facilities;
▶ appropriate educational provision geared to the child's special educational needs;
▶ advice guidance and counselling;
▶ family aides, particularly if the main carer is ill;
▶ day care with a childminder, or in a playgroup or nursery;
▶ respite care in which children are cared for in a residential setting;
▶ specific medical care and attention tuned to the child's physical or mental health problems causing or arising out of the severe challenging behaviour;
▶ leisure activities.

Under the provisions of the Children Act (1989) and certainly in tune with its philosophy, the various agencies confronted by the challenge of children with learning disabilities and severe challenging behaviour should never seek or contemplate removal of a child from the family home, unless all the services which could possibly be provided have been provided and the child's family is still unable to cope. Regrettably, from the evidence presented to the Committee, this was far from the case. Since few local authority areas possessed good quality local services within their own boundaries, many of the approaches identified, involved sending children to residential schools out of the area or to totally inappropriate local provision not geared to this group's specific needs.

A good example of a service being provided under s.17 of the Children Act (1989) is the provision of respite care. Such provision fulfils the duty to provide a service appropriate to the needs of this group of children. If respite carers can be found for this group of children, they provided a much needed support for families and an invaluable break from, the constant demands of the child with learning disabilities who also presents severe challenging behaviour.

Where respite care is provided in residential children homes, then the (amended) Children's Homes Regulations 1991 and the DoH Guidance on Permissible Forms of Control in Children Residential Care would be applicable. Where respite care is provided by specially approved foster carers then they would be subject to the guidelines laid down in the Foster Placement (Children) Regulations 1991 (also amended).

7.2.4 Reviews and complaints procedures

Guidance issued pursuant to the Children Act (1989) made it clear where there was any 'significant involvement' with a family then reviews of such involvement should take place at regular intervals (DoH, 1991b: para 2.10). Where, pursuant to the provisions of Section 20, the service of accommodation is provided to a family, then the responsible authority ie the local authority, voluntary organisation or person carrying on a home must comply with Regulations. The Guidance (DoH 1991e) states, that:

> 'any meeting which is convened for the purpose of considering the child's case ... falls within these Regulations. Whether such a meeting is called a planning meeting or a review or a review meeting will not determine whether it is in fact part of a review. This will depend upon the purpose for which the meeting is convened.'

Under these Regulations which, as has been indicated, apply when a child is being provided with the service of accommodation under s.20, reviews must take place within four weeks of accommodation being provided, then within three months of the first review and subsequently at six monthly intervals. As has been indicated, the Guidance issued in Volume 2 further indicates the desirability of holding comparable reviews wherever there is significant involvement with the family in the way of providing a range of support services.

From evidence given to the Committee, it is clear that reviewing of all the arrangements relating to services being provided to children with learning disabilities who also present severe challenging behaviour, is often infrequently done, poorly coordinated and often leads to an inefficient deployment of resources from amongst the agencies concerned.

In addition, many giving evidence to the Committee and particularly those involved with special provision, commented on the changing nature of personnel at reviews, especially those held on children placed out of county or out of local authority boundaries. This problem is not restricted to residential placements made out of the local authority area. It is even more likely to be experienced by families who seek support services and who are subject to ever-changing personnel on their children's cases. The quality of such reviews is also something which gives rise to considerable concern. Very often they appear to concentrate on very mundane matters rather than on the major issues of whether the services being provided are actually the right ones or whether changes are needed in order to achieve a better outcome for the child and the family. This is particularly important in relation to children with learning disabilities and severe challenging behaviour.

Where reviews are not required by the Regulations because they are concerned with the provision of services rather than family placements, then extra efforts should be made to ensure the regularity of such reviews in order to improve the efficient deployment of resources. The format of such reviews should nevertheless follow closely that laid down for the statutory reviews. Thus there should be proper preparation, an agenda set, the most appropriate people invited and a suitable venue chosen. For the statutory reviews, the Regulations require the responsible authority to seek out and take into account the views of the child, the parents, any person with parental responsibility and others whose views are considered relevant and those persons should be invited to meetings and notified of decisions.

Under the Statutory Reviews the Guidance indicates (DoH, 1991c: para 8.15) that children and parents may need to attend separate parts of a Review or children may need a friendly supporter. In many cases it is obviously difficult for children with learning disabilities and severe challenging behaviour to be given a proper opportunity to participate in reviews of services being provided to them and their families. Nevertheless, it is vitally important that the child is accorded respect for his or her position and that, as far as possible, the child's feelings about the services which are being provided are identified to the review. There are all sorts of ways in which children communicate their feelings about the services they are experiencing and it is not as difficult as some people imply, to identify those aspects of the services of which they approve and those they dislike.

Whilst the Children Act (1989) in s.26(3) does provide for the establishment of representation procedures by local authorities, many families commented in evidence to the Committee that they really had neither the time nor the energy to access such procedures in order to make representations or complaints about services they were or were not receiving. Everyone needs to recognise that looking after a child with learning disabilities and severe challenging behaviour is a 24 hour job for most families and that it is difficult, if not impossible, to envisage taking time out to make a complaint using the rather cumbersome procedures established pursuant to the Children Act (1989). Nevertheless, it is possible for people to complain, not only about particular services, but also about the failure to make provision for services. Indeed, families may wish to complain that their child has not been classified as a child in need and if a local authority does refuse to consider that a child is a child in need, then the appropriate remedy may be by way of judicial review. The regulations and the statutory provisions provide for an independent element to be included within the representations procedure, but as has already been indicated, most felt that the procedures were too cumbersome to access in their particular circumstances.

7.2.5 Cooperation between authorities

There are provisions in the Children Act (1989), the Education Act (1996) and the relevant health services legislation requiring cooperation between the various agencies who might be involved in providing support to families of children with learning disabilities and severe challenging behaviour. Thus under s.27 of the Children Act (1989), where it appears to a local authority that any other local authority, LEA, local housing authority, health authority or NHS Trust or any other person so authorised, could assist with the provision of services for any child, then the authority whose help is so requested must comply with such a request, if it is shown to be compatible with their own statutory or other duties and does not unduly prejudice the discharge of any of their functions.

Specifically, s.27(4) provides that every local authority shall assist any LEA with the provision of services for any child within the local authority area who has special educational needs. Whilst the Children Act (1989) is primarily directed at Social services departments, s.27 acknowledges that the services which may be required by such groups as children with learning disabilities and severe challenging behaviour are also the responsibility of a range of agencies.

Even when issuing its own guidance, the government was aware that families of children with special needs might be being shunted back and forth between different departments or authorities. In the statutory Code of Guidance for Local Authorities on Homelessness (HMSO 1991), it was noted that:

'each department and authority has a responsibility to those who approach it under its own relevant legislation. However, a corporate policy and clear procedures in respect of collaboration … will help to ensure cooperation at all levels (para 6.16).'

Unfortunately, as has been identified, families of children with learning disabilities who also present severe challenging behaviour did not experience a well coordinated corporate policy approach to their problems. The Committee heard that, sometimes, there could be a wide range of service inputs or, conversely, a total lack of provision, both arising from a lack of coordination and cooperation.

Section 28 of the Children Act (1989) further imposes duties on local authorities to consult the appropriate educational authority before accommodating a child at an establishment which provides education, inform them of the placement and tell them when it ends. This provision applies to placements in boarding schools and homes which are also schools.

Correspondingly, under s.322 of the Education Act (1996), a duty is imposed on health authorities and local authorities to help and assist LEAs in the identification and assessment of children with special educational needs. All the children with learning disabilities and severe challenging behaviour fall into this category.

7.3 Legislative provision in Scotland and Northern Ireland

The Committee has concentrated primarily on the problems affecting this group of children as manifested in England and Wales. The Children Act (1989) only applies to England and Wales, but Scotland and Northern Ireland now have separate legislation and procedures which bring them broadly into line with provision made for children in England and Wales. Thus, the law on the care and upbringing of children in Northern Ireland is moving into line with England and Wales. A commencement order brought into operation the main provisions of the Children (Northern Ireland) Order 1995 from 4th November 1996. The law and particularly that relating to the provision of services to children in need, will be substantially similar to that pertaining in England and Wales. Legislation in Scotland, namely the Children (Scotland) Act 1995 also provides for a broadly similar regime to operate in Scotland, particularly as it affects the promotion of the welfare of children in need and the provision of services particularly to children with disabilities and to others described as being in need under the statutory provisions.

Other legal issues

7.4 Background to issues of care, control and safety

Implementation of the Children Act (1989) has stimulated a growing debate about the quality of care for children with learning disabilities and challenging behaviour and the legal basis for a range of treatments and interventions, particularly those involving the use of control and restraint. Although the Act has highlighted many concerns about children's residential and day services in general, specific difficulties have been encountered in services used by children with challenging behaviour.

There is general agreement that future policy and practice must be in accordance with the legal framework of the Children Act (1989) and that policies must reflect the sound child-care principles on which the Act is based. The issues are complex and raise significant dilemmas for which there are no simple solutions.

The Mental Health Foundation recognised the need for urgent information on the legal implications of the Children Act (1989) for children with learning disabilities and challenging behaviour and set up a working party to oversee a Research Project led by Professor Christina Lyon which resulted in the publication of two reports on legal issues arising from the care, control and safety of children with learning disabilities who also present severe challenging behaviour:

▶ a policy and guidance document (Lyon, 1994a), referred to here as Policy and Guidance; and
▶ a guide for parents and carers (1994b), referred to here as the Parents and Carers Guide.

We have referred readers to sections of her reports, where we thought it would be helpful. Many of the issues which these reports address were echoed in evidence we received from parents and carers, as well as from purchasers and providers. We have also drawn on information obtained during the Foundation's dissemination of Professor Lyon's work. This confirmed the Committee's view that there is currently considerable uncertainty about the legal basis for the care, control and treatment of children with severe challenging behaviour amongst purchasers, providers and families.

After some general comments about the dilemmas facing parents, carers and professionals, the existing legal framework and the principles from which legal issues should be approached, we focus on three broad areas which were reflected in the evidence we received:

▶ parental responsibility and the provision of care, control and safety;
▶ control and restraint;
▶ medical treatment and consent.

7.5 Challenges and dilemmas

'It's when I take Judy [age 12] out that it all goes wrong. She is fine until something upsets her then she scratches and bites; she nearly bit an old man the other day. He had a black hat and she doesn't like black hats! My sister said, why not sew the sleeves of her coat together, because she is like a windmill. I did it, but they didn't like it at school when I told them. What's more like abuse: locked up all the time or going out for a walk with your sleeves sewn up?'

'Daniel [age 12] is held down or tied up most of the time. Sounds like a gangster film, doesn't it? Sometimes we use special clothes that restrain his hands and we tie him into the buggy major. I have a lovely big red woollen scarf to do that with. It looks okay too. Of course he doesn't need a buggy but we couldn't face outings otherwise. We keep hoping he'll improve. But we have a social worker now. She is really nice but she tells us we can't tie Daniel up like this. I think she talked about the UN Convention or something. I think Daniel has got a right to be restrained. He will be locked up if he is not kept in order. What can parents do when all the professionals have failed?'

Parents (as well as professionals) provided clear and compelling evidence of the very real dilemmas facing families and other carers on a daily – and in some cases hour-by-hour – basis, as they sought to provide children with the best possible care while also trying to offer them as normal a lifestyle as possible.

'Clearer legal guidelines for children with challenging behaviour and learning disabilities would give staff greater confidence in dealing with and managing these behaviours. Too often staff complain that guidance is rather clearer on non-permissible actions than [on how to deal] with real situations. Many behaviours are very violent and persistent. They risk injury to the child, peers, staff and members of the public. They lead to many dilemmas such as deciding on the interests of the group which may be different from the interests of individual members. On the spot decisions are often difficult and dilemmas exist such as 'Do I take a child out who sometimes has challenging behaviour?' What about risk of injury to the public? Do we have an option to prevent someone from having a community experience due to their challenging behaviour?' (Head of Care, National Autistic Society school)

The particular dilemmas for each child's carers will vary as the experiences of Judy and Daniel (see above) and Mark and Mary (see below) and their carers illustrate, but some occur frequently and raise important and difficult issues:

- How do you balance the needs of an individual child with challenging behaviour with the needs (eg for safety) of other children?
- How do you resolve the situation when formal and informal carers have conflicting ideas about how a particular child's need for care and control should be met?
- What action, if any, can be taken when a service excludes a child with challenging behaviour, because staff are uncertain about the legality of using restraints or other types of procedures, or feel they are not competent to manage the challenging behaviour?
- Can a decision taken by one statutory agency be legally challenged by another service and/or the family?
- What action, if any, can be taken when an intervention which has been successful in managing challenging behaviour has to be stopped because someone has challenged the legality of the situation?
- Is it legally permissible to physically restrain a child so that they can go out into the community without endangering their own and others' safety and can thus lead a more normal life?

7.6 The current legal framework for care, control and safety

Uncertainties about the legal framework have potentially harmful consequences for the development of child-centred, appropriate and more inclusive services for children with challenging behaviour.

'The Children Act (1989) did not address the needs of children with disabilities who also present severe challenging behaviour and limited the response Social services departments could make. There is too much emphasis on desirability rather than specific statutory responsibility. It has also created further difficulties for carers in terms of no clearly defined guidelines for issues such as 'restraint' procedures – parents are now unsure what is 'lawful' under child protection systems and what isn't.' (Parent's organisation, supported by and based at NHS trust hospital)

'The Children Act (1989) and discussion of issues around care, control and treatment did not demonstrate an awareness of the existence of children with severe challenging behaviour and learning disabilities.' (Child and adolescent psychiatrist)

The Committee is extremely concerned that misunderstandings about the Act have emerged in the evidence we received. The introduction of the Children Act (1989) rightly led many professionals, parents and informal carers of children with challenging behaviour to review their care practices. But one unfortunate outcome has been the growth of a series of myths about what the Children Act (1989) supposedly 'allows' or 'forbids'.

Misunderstandings have arisen, often based on individual beliefs rather than on what the law actually says, although there have been attempts to legitimise particular viewpoints by vague references to 'fundamental human rights'. What many people have failed to realise is that the Children Act (1989) makes no specific mention of children with learning disabilities and challenging behaviour. Neither do the associated guidelines which have subsequently appeared.

In the DoH guidelines on permissible forms of control in residential care (1993), for example, children with learning disabilities only are mentioned, but then too briefly. There is no specific guidance on dealing with children with learning disabilities and challenging behaviour and the guidance is mainly about dealing with children of normal capacities who exhibit what could be termed 'more usual' challenging behaviour.

Similarly, circular 9/94 on the 'Education of Children with Emotional and Behavioural Difficulties' (Department of Education, 1994) makes no specific reference to children with learning disabilities and challenging behaviour, although it does make some useful points about issues such as the use of specialist services and the application of controls and sanctions (see para 115) in a section headed 'Other Issues'.

Within the laws of England, Wales, Northern Ireland and Scotland there are a number of legislative provisions which seek to comply with the demands set by the UN Convention on the rights of the child. Article 23 provides that states which have ratified the Convention recognise that

> 'mentally or physically disabled child should enjoy a full and decent life in conditions which ensure dignity, promote self reliance and facilitate the child's active participation in the community'

The Children Act (1989) was hailed in England and Wales as a fundamentally important piece of legislation dealing with children in that it sought to introduce what many saw as a comprehensive and comprehensible civil legal framework to deal with all children regardless of their particular circumstances. Nevertheless, special provision was made for those children deemed to be 'in need', as has been seen above.

7.7 Basic principles governing the care of children

Any service (or individual) seeking to provide for the care, control and safety of a child with learning disabilities and challenging behaviour must consider the particular needs of that individual child. Inevitably, the functional abilities and competence of the child will partly determine the appropriate response to the severe challenging behaviour, but that response must also respect the importance of ensuring that services reflect established child care principles.

The Committee strongly supports the principles set out in Professor Lyon's reports (1994a, 1994b) that:

- ▶ each child must be accorded respect for their rights as an individual;
- ▶ any response to a child's behaviour must be based on a consideration of what is in that child's best interests and what they would recognise themselves as being in their own interests, were they of the age and capacity to make such decisions themselves;
- ▶ the child's welfare must be the paramount consideration;
- ▶ all reasonable steps must be taken to promote and safeguard the child's welfare.

7.8 Parental responsibility: provision of care, control and safety

> Policy and Guidance: pp. 29-42
>
> Parents and Carers Guide: pp. 7-9

In considering the care, control and safety of children with learning disabilities and challenging behaviour, two concepts are central: 'parental responsibility' and the 'paramount interests of the child'.

The notion of parental responsibility is one of the pivotal concepts of the Children Act (1989) and the Children (Northern Ireland) Order 1995, replacing the concept of 'rights' and, in the words of the Lord Chancellor (P&G: 31), acknowledging that 'the overwhelming purpose of parenthood is the responsibility for caring for/and raising the child to be a properly developed adult both physically and morally'.

The Children Act (1989) directs that courts in England and Wales must give paramount consideration to the child's welfare. (A similar provision is found in s.3 of the Northern Irish law and s.16 of the Scottish legislation.) Thus parents of children with learning disabilities and challenging behaviour (as well as carers and professionals) must always consider whether their actions will be in the paramount interests of the child.

Parents may also delegate care of a child, although this does not mean they relinquish their own responsibility. Those acting in loco parentis may include a range of professionals and care staff in residential or day settings such as schools, other staff in those establishments such as cleaners, catering staff and minibus drivers, through to health-care professionals who may be looking after a child on a short or long-term basis because the child requires a particular treatment or intervention.

Substitute carers of children with learning disabilities and challenging behaviour would be expected:

▶ to do all that a responsible parent would do; and

▶ all that would be necessary to protect the child; and

▶ to take whatever actions may be necessary to prevent the child harming himself or others or exposing himself or others, to harm.

A clear understanding of these fundamental concepts of parental responsibility, acting in the paramount interests of the child and doing what is reasonable to safeguard and promote the welfare of the child is essential if parents and other carers are to be able to understand their actions and explain them to others.

7.9 Control and restraint

'Fourteen-year-old Mary beats her head with her fists; she has already blinded herself in the left eye and the right one is developing cataracts. Our physiotherapist has had some splints made which stop Mary bending her arms and we tether her wrists to the arms of her wheelchair. I suspect we may be doing the wrong thing since reading guidelines about the Children Act (1989). What should we be doing to be sure we are not breaking the law?'

> See also:
>
> Policy and Guidance: Parts III and VI
>
> Parents and Carers Guide: pp. 20-27, 31-37.

Because of the nature of some of the interventions used with children who have learning disabilities and challenging behaviour, protection from abuse is of paramount importance with these particularly vulnerable children. It is equally important however, to understand that the Mental Health Foundation work on legal issues is not seeking to legitimise unacceptable methods of control and restraint. Rather, the aim is to provide constructive guidance on interpreting current legislation in England and Wales in order to assist parents and professionals faced with real-life situations requiring varied responses to the care and control of vulnerable children.

The Committee endorses this approach. Both the reports (Lyon 1994a, 1994b) analyse the justifications which might be used by someone who has used control or restraint, but also make it clear that these should never be put forward as mere excuses or used to justify the illegitimate use of restraint.

It is essential that we understand the context in which control and restraint may be used by professionals, carers and parents. Everyone needs to be aware of this, whether they are someone with a position of authority in services or an ordinary member of the community.

Most people have no direct experience of severe challenging behaviour and so may fail to fully understand the problems and dilemmas which families and care staff actually face. Without direct experience, we may also fail to grasp why particular strategies may ultimately have to be adopted to ensure that a child's welfare is safeguarded. Stating categorically, for example, that restraint should never be used may not be in the child's best interests. A great deal more training is required on what the law actually provides in this area for those such as Inspection Unit staff, who may only infrequently come into contact with families or carers having to adopt such strategies.

The Policy and Guidance and Parents and Carers Guide (Lyon a, 1994) contain detailed guidance about control and restraint and those seeking further guidance are recommended to refer to them. We set out here what we see as the overarching principles which should be borne in mind when restraint and control measures are being considered:

▶ Restrictive measures should only be adopted to deal with severe challenging behaviour when there is no alternative and should be used in the least detrimental manner and for the shortest or possible time. They should never be used a result of pressures on staff or because of staff shortages as a matter of convenience.

▶ Any measures of control, whether used in the child's family home or in other settings, should always be part of an individual care plan and should first have been discussed by the parents, professionals and carers concerned.

▶ Plans which include use of control or restraint should be regularly reviewed and re-assessed in the light of the child's responses and reactions to the measures which have been adopted.

The experiences of Mary (see above), who repeatedly tore at her eyes, vividly demonstrates the extremely fine line between protecting a child from abuse by others (through inappropriate restraint) and protecting them from the incredibly harmful (and permanent) consequences of their own actions. No parent or carer would wish to restrain a child, but if the alternative is that the child ends up totally blind, parents or carers may equally fear that they could be deemed negligent for having failed to take proper care of the child by seeking to restrain her self-injurious actions.

Mark's experiences demonstrate graphically that even where control or restraint are part of an agreed plan, actions may be questioned:

'Mark is a large fifteen-year-old who has been very violent in the past and continues to be so unless handled in a consistent, firm yet sympathetic manner. He has some language, understands simple cause and effect, recognises when he is likely to be violent and can rôle play more appropriate strategies he might have used to deal with the anger-provoking situation once he is calm. Whilst at residential school he was taught to go to his room when his anger was aroused and there he was provided with materials he could rip up – a method which successfully discharged his anger. Once calm, staff talked him through what had happened and got him to suggest and rôle play how he might have handled the situation better.

In the early days of this programme, staff took him to his room when he became angry and he was instructed how to discharge his anger and the door was closed. If he attempted to leave his room before calming, he was told to return and the door would be held closed. If he struggled to open it it would be locked. Mark was never left. Two staff remained outside the room and observed his behaviour through the one-way panel. They rewarded any diminution in his angry behaviour with encouraging, calming comments. All such incidents were fully recorded. Mark's parents, his local authority educational psychologist and social worker were fully aware of the programme and had endorsed its use in writing. They were all delighted with Mark's progress under the programme.

Senior officers of Mark's local authority disagreed with the programme on the grounds that this liberty was being restricted – as set out in the Children Act (1989). Mark was eventually excluded from school because his behaviour became unmanageable when use of his room was precluded (on the instruction of the local authority). The serious injuries to staff simply could not be accepted. Following abortive attempts to support Mark at home he was briefly placed in a social services facility, from which he walked out. After a brief, violent and destructive period at home his parents were told to exclude him on the advice of social services staff. He was immediately arrested and imprisoned overnight by the local police, before being brought to court, admitted into a secure unit under a 18-day section under the 1983 Mental Health Act where he was heavily sedated.

Were the successful, carefully planned, precisely conducted and continuously monitored procedures used at the school really illegal? Did the local authority's senior administrative staff have the legal right to terminate a humane and demonstrably efficacious teaching procedure which had been thoroughly worked out and had multi-agency agreement and clinically approval? Could the local authority's decision be legally challenged?'

In considering the criminal and civil law implications, therefore, we recognise that parents' and carers' actions may at times be called into question by others, even when those actions are being carried out as part of an agreed care plan. Mark's experiences demonstrate this all too clearly. What ultimately happened to Mark cannot be deemed to have been in his best interests. Yet we should also have due respect to Mark's rights as an individual when seeking to provide for his care, control and safety.

A balance has to be struck between the child being restrained and the person doing the restraining. If less harm is caused either to the child or to others by the use of restraint, then such restraint is likely to be deemed reasonable. However, each situation has to be judged separately, bearing in mind the needs of each individual child.

7.10 Relevant government departmental guidance

Professor Lyon's two documents (1994a, 1994b) explore in great detail and with great care a whole range of guidance which has been issued by government departments and which may be of possible relevance to the parent, carers and educators of children with learning disabilities who also present severe challenging behaviour. Whilst it is impossible to reproduce the analysis in which Professor Lyon engages in these two documents, the sort of problems with which they purport to deal might usefully be highlighted here.

The Department of Education's circular on pupils with emotional and behavioural problems (DFE, 1994), under the heading 'other issues', a number of useful points are made:

- The pupil's age, understanding and any disability he or she may have will need to be taken into account in determining the appropriate sanction to be applied (para 110).

- On occasions there is no alternative to restraining pupils physically in their own and others' interests (para 115), for example, if they are seriously damaging property, or committing some criminal act which risks harm to people or property (para 115).

- In such instances no more than the minimum force necessary should be used, taking into account all the circumstances (para 115).

- Such interventions should be positive and made only when they are likely to succeed (para 115).

- Desirably more than one adult should be present (though this is not always possible) (para 115).

- It is wholly inappropriate to use corporal punishment for children with emotional and behavioural difficulties and it is illegal for all publicly funded pupils (para 112).

The DoH (1993) has also issued Guidance on 'permissible forms for control in children's residential care'. It was designed to cover young people living in children's homes, rather than schools, but offers positive and practical advice to staff on the care and control of young people with normal capacities living in residential accommodation. Part 8 - 'How the age understanding and competence of a child can bear on appropriate methods of control' - might be looked to for guidance when dealing with children with learning disabilities who also present severe challenging behaviour. S8.3 provides that:

'children of any age may have an impaired ability to recognise and understand danger. This may, for example, be because of serious learning disabilities, autism or severe emotional disorder. For such children there may be need to take action including the use of physical restraint and the need for physical intervention may be more frequent.'

The Guidance further states that brief periods of withdrawal away from the group into a calming environment may be more effective for a severely agitated child than holding or physical restraint. (It should also be pointed out that this mirrors very closely the guidance provided in the DFE circular 9/94.) Indeed, parents giving evidence to Professor Lyon's working party pointed out that in relation to autistic children, the use of holding or the application of physical restraint might result in an exacerbation of their challenging behaviour. Paragraph 8.4 of the DoH (1993) guidance advises that in homes which look after such children there will be a particular need to ensure that children do not have unsupervised access to unsafe areas including outside the house or grounds. The safety of the child is said to be 'important'. It suggests that homes should adopt normal domestic approaches to security, including, for example, the locking of all external doors at night. The guidance also advises that the reasonable application of these practices would not constitute a restriction of liberty.

The Committee believes that the Guidance given by the DFE (1994) and the DoH (1993) is very important for all those involved in the care of this group of children and that much greater training on law should be provided to Inspection Unit staff, managers of children's homes, those running schools, day centres and health care establishments and further, that advice and training should also be sought from professionals in the psychiatric area who may be able to advise on a source of training in respect of safe methods of restraining children and young people. Indeed, the DoH Guidance states in s.11 that managers should satisfy themselves that training is relevant and appropriate and that it is part of a programme which puts use within the full context of care and control in residential child care. Such advice could equally be directed across the whole range of those looking after this group of children.

7.11 Medical treatment

> See also:
>
> Policy and Guidance: pp. 149-77
>
> Parents and Carers Guide: pp. 43-49

The issue of medical treatment is challenging and may involve substantial misuse or even, at times, serious abuse. Careful and holistic assessment is crucial and all treatments and interventions, including the use of medication, must be constantly questioned, evaluated, reviewed and, where necessary, reformulated.

To avoid polarisations between medical and social models of care, health and social care agencies must work closely together. The legal basis for this is s27 of the Children Act (1989) which lays a duty on the local authority and the health authority to assist each other in the discharge of their legal duties and responsibilities towards children 'in need' – including children with disabilities.

In some instances, medication may be used as part of a long-term treatment programme. Appropriately administered, medication can bring about a radical improvement in behaviour – not by sedating the child so that he or she no longer causes problems, but by accurately assessing and treating underlying potential physical problems so that the child's behaviour improves.

In other cases, medication may have to be administered in an emergency, as a last resort and where the child's health or well-being is threatened.

The Policy and Guidance and the Parents and Carers Guide both address in detail the complex issues relating to consent, eg whether a child with learning disabilities and challenging behaviour can consent to treatment.

7.12 Key principles

The Committee believes in the following:

▶ Focused, targeted and properly planned coordination of the delivery of services to children with learning disabilities who also present severe challenging behaviour and their families

▶ Focused, targeted and properly prepared reviews of the provision of such services

▶ Tightening up of the legal provisions requiring such cooperation and coordination and removal of the clause which allows authorities to escape from complying with requests for assistance with other authorities if such is not consistent with their own statutory duties.

▶ Proper resourcing of services required to be delivered under the legislative provisions.

▶ Properly training on and awareness of the Guidance on Law relating to control and restraint measures published by the Mental Health Foundation in 1994.

Recommendations

▶ Section 27 of the Children Act (1989), which requires cooperation and coordination between different agencies should be clarified and strengthened. Local and health authorities should not retain their current power to refuse to comply with requests for assistance from other authorities if they consider that such requests are not consistent with their own statutory duties.

▶ As indicated in this chapter, the Children Act (1989) provides a clear legal framework for the provision of services for children who are regarded as being 'in need' or who are disabled. We recommend that central and local government should urgently address the resourcing of such services and, in particular, the funding mechanisms to support children who have complex and therefore expensive special needs.

▶ Information and training relating to the law on control and restraint as set out in the Mental Health Foundation's guidance (Lyon 1994a, 1994b) should be made available for all staff working with children with learning disabilities and severe challenging behaviour. Such information and training should be provided for staff working in all three statutory services and within any providers in the voluntary or independent sectors.

▶ Local and health authorities should ensure that area child protection committees and local child protection services have appropriate information and training with regard to the legal basis for permissible control and treatment.

References

Children's Rights Development Group (1994). The UK Agenda for Children. CRDU.

Department of Health (1991a) the Children Act (1989) Guidance and Regulations Volume 6 Children with Disabilities. HMSO.

DoH (1991b) the Children Act (1989) Guidance and Regulations Volume 2 Family Support Day Care and Educational Provision for Young Children. HMSO.

DoH (1991c) the Children Act (1989) Guidance and Regulations Volume 3 Family Placements. HMSO.

DoH (1993) Guidance on Permissible Forms of Control in Children's Residential Care Circular. LAC (93)13.

Department of Education (1994) Education of Children with Emotional and Behavioural Difficulties. DFE Circular 9/94.

HMSO (1994) The UK's First Report to the UN Committee on the Rights of the Child. HMSO.

Lyon Christina (1994a) Legal issues arising from the care control and safety of children with learning disabilities who also present severe challenging behaviour: Policy and Guidance. Mental Health Foundation.

Lyon Christina (1994b) Legal issues arising from the care and control of children with learning disabilities who also present severe challenging behaviour: A Guide for Parents and Carers. Mental Health Foundation.

CHAPTER 8
Commissioning and purchasing in the health service: assessment and planning in social services

In this chapter, both the rôle of the health service and the assessment and planning functions of local authority social service departments are considered. However, from the outset it is important to emphasise that both agencies need to develop a shared vision and joint planning for children with learning disabilities and severe challenging behaviour.

Commissioning and purchasing in the health service

In the first part of this chapter we have sought to summarise the current collective knowledge, ideas and experiences of a number of experts in the field of commissioning and purchasing across the country. Purchasing and commissioning specifically for children with learning disabilities and severe challenging behaviour is still in its infancy and as yet we do not know a great deal about how best to proceed. However, we have been able to draw on work in services such as child and adolescent mental health which has direct relevance to the children who are our concern here.

8.1 Principles

All commissioning and purchasing should be based on, and take account, of the following:

- Children with learning disabilities and severe challenging behaviour are not a homogeneous group.
- There are many different causes of disability and of behavioural difficulties.
- The needs of each child will be different and services should offer an individualised response.
- Children with learning disabilities and severe challenging behaviour have complex needs which require specialist services.
- Specialist help should be available within a continuum of services which are provided for all children and which may be used by any child.
- Children with learning disabilities and severe challenging behaviour have continuing, often lifelong, needs for special support.
- Special needs in other family members will often be generated by children with learning disabilities and severe challenging behaviour; meeting these needs can enable the family to remain closely involved in the care of the disabled child.

8.2 The Current situation

The commissioning and purchasing of services for children with learning disabilities and challenging behaviour will need to address a number of shortcomings in service provision currently facing these children and their families.

Children with learning disabilities and challenging behaviour often have difficulty in accessing ordinary primary health care and health promotion facilities such as dental and vision checks. If they become ill, there can be problems with gaining access to secondary care.

Nationwide, there is a shortage of learning disability services specifically for children.

Individual paediatricians sometimes take a special interest in this field or may work in collaboration with adult learning disability services, but the level of expertise is extremely limited in many localities. In addition, mental health services with specialist expertise in children with learning disabilities are a scarce resource.

Because of the shortage of specialist services such as these in most parts of the country, children with challenging behaviour tend to be offered one-off interventions, often in response to a crisis. Unless the need for long-term preventative and continuing input is clearly acknowledged, appropriate provision will not be developed.

'Any disability in a family will usually mean extra support in day-to-day living arrangements. But no one seems interested in support. It's all crisis intervention and you get your points for breaking down.' (A parent)

The extent to which health, education, social services and other local authority services are required will vary according to the needs of each child and will change over time. The health service is most often the first to be involved in the diagnosis of a child with developmental delay and learning disabilities and in decisions about management. Later the health service again will probably be the source of specialist help for emotional and behavioural difficulties, should they occur. But initial concern may first be raised in the education system and education will certainly be of major importance throughout childhood (see Chapter 4). A requirement for support from social services tends to increase as a child grows up. However, children with learning disabilities and severe challenging behaviour will be children 'in need' under the Children Act (1989) (see Chapter 7). As such, social services are the lead agency in obtaining services and the health authority has a duty to provide appropriate medical, nursing and therapeutic services. Everyone in the system has a partial view except the child or young person themselves.

The Audit Commission (1994) noted evidence of poor joint commissioning and joint individual assessment arrangements for children with a wide range of disabilities, commenting that only 25 per cent of the parents consulted felt that services were well coordinated. The Commission also expressed concern at the lack of clear criteria for assessment for particular levels of service input for an individual child.

'The professionals don't agree amongst themselves. You get caught in the cross-fire. We all want what is best for our children.' (A parent)

It is essential that children with the complex and continuing needs of those with learning disabilities and severe challenging behaviour are included in strategic planning (commissioning) in the health service and similarly in local authority children's services planning and that agencies jointly agree the required input for individual children, regardless of which agency has identified the need for services or which agency will pay the bill.

8.3 Challenges for specialist services

Highly specialised services are expensive and also tend to be an 'occasional' service which a health district may or may not use in any one year. As a result, these specialist services may or may not be purchased on a regular basis and are in danger of becoming decimated due to lack of consistent reliable funding. They cannot maintain their resources nor undertake important innovative work. This in turn can lead to low staff morale.

A recent review of child and adolescent mental health services (Williams and Richardson 1995) raised various concerns about the provision of highly specialised services and their relationship to other specialist services. These concerns are equally applicable to specialist services for children with learning disabilities and severe challenging behaviour. (see page 70)

8.4 Guidance on commissioning and purchasing of specialist services

Two sets of relevant guidance on specialist services have been published recently by the NHS Management Executive in 1993 and in 1995 by the British Paediatric Association (BPA) (Verrier Jones and Lissauer, 1995).

The BPA (Verrier Jones and Lissauer, 1995) rightly places the child and family at the centre of the organisational network of services that interface with specialist paediatric tertiary care. (see figure 8.1 on age 71)

Concerns about the provision of very specialised services

- Difficulties in their relationships with local children's primary and secondary health care services:
  - difficulties of liaison with referrers;
  - difficulties of discharge planning;
  - disinclination to share specialist skills and secondary services.
- The vulnerability of very specialised services in the internal market:
  - lack of contracts for services creates difficulties in financial and service planning;
  - financial insecurity hampers development of new services and restricts their capacity to disseminate specialist skills
- Inappropriate use of very specialised services when they are found to be providing less specialised interventions in districts with under-developed secondary care services.
- Inappropriate use of local services to provide more specialised care:
  - eg non-use of very specialised services on grounds of their cost or insufficient capacity, can lead to disruption of local children's secondary care services through disproportionate time and effort spent on difficult or extremely challenging cases.
- Poor systems of quality control and performance monitoring: – the absence of commissioning mechanisms often results in very specialised services not being subject to questions on monitoring of their activity, effectiveness and efficiency.

The report sets out detailed guidance including recommended staffing levels for many of the paediatric sub-specialties. However, apart from paediatric neurology, no guidance is given on the psychiatry of learning disability in children or for other specialist requirements in this field such as clinical psychologists or therapists. There are no data upon which to base estimates of the cost of a comprehensive service for children with learning disabilities and severe challenging behaviour.

Ensuring that children and families have access to specialist provision as part of a continuum of children's services must be seen as a priority and the Committee would like to draw attention to the guidance on how best to undertake this aspect of planning, included in Together We Stand (Williams and Richardson, 1995)

Figure 8.2 on page 71 provides a visual conception of an idealised integrated service. In this, the contributions of the main sectors of care and the needs for services of a range of capabilities and specialisations, are drawn together with the facilities for reciprocal consultation, training, support and advice in a three-dimensional model (NHS/HAS 1995)

8.5 Commissioning and purchasing rôles

Commissioning is the comprehensive framework within which purchasing takes place. It is strategic and involves defining, managing and monitoring the market. It is an iterative process based on the assessment of population needs for health services.

Purchasing refers to the various technical procedures carried out by purchasers in order to secure and monitor the services they are buying from providers. It includes contracting – the mechanism by which services are purchased based on specification of the service required to meet needs.

Health authorities are responsible for commissioning in the health service. They also undertake a limited amount of direct purchasing, generally for the more specialised services.

GP fundholders are significant direct purchasers. It is important that they are involved in strategic commissioning decisions.

Health and local authorities have somewhat different approaches to purchasing and commissioning. Local authorities are responsible for care management and are required to purchase packages of care for individuals, whereas health authorities buy sectors of care for the population. Individual assessments are part of the local authority's purchasing rôle but in the health service these are usually the provider's responsibility.

Fig 8.1 Relationships between primary, secondary and tertiary care for children and their families

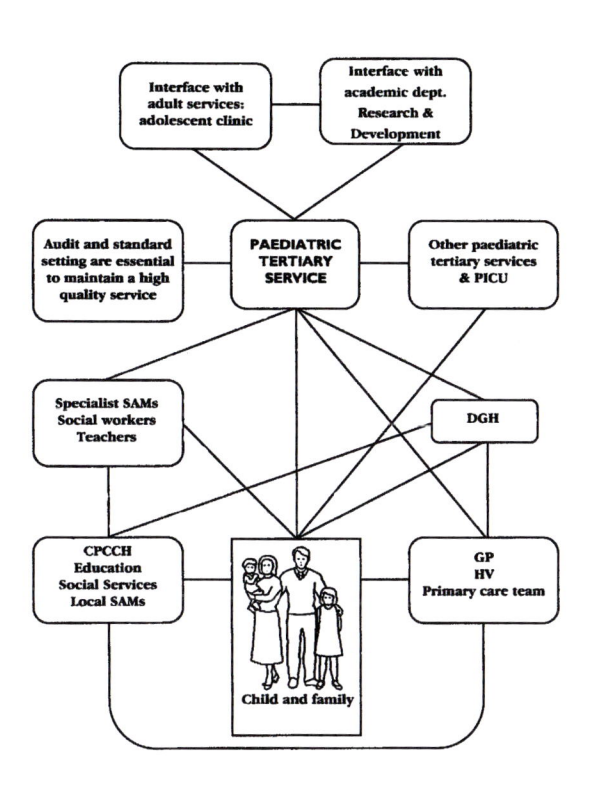

Source: Verrier, Jones And Lissauer, 1995, The Royal College of Paediatrics and Child Health

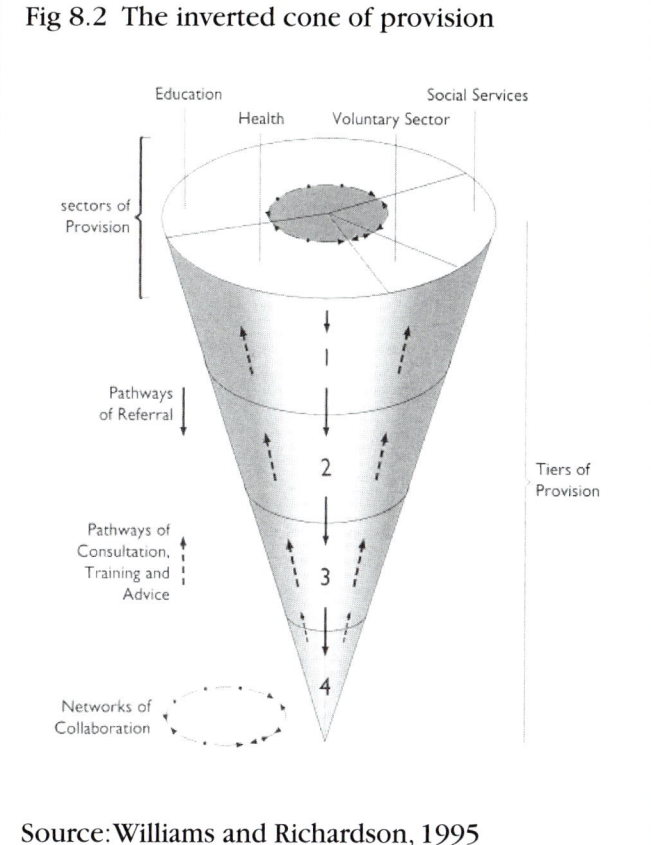

Fig 8.2 The inverted cone of provision

Source: Williams and Richardson, 1995

Crown Copyright is Reproduced with the permission of the Controller of Her Majesty's Stationery Office

8.6 Developing an informed approach

Our understanding of children with learning disabilities and severe challenging behaviour and our experience of providing services to them is growing all the time but the knowledge and expertise is held by different professional groups and is differently available in different parts of the country. It is essential that commissioning decisions are made on the best and most comprehensive current information. Too many people with a major stake in commissioning services still have little understanding of the issues. Despite the difficulties inherent in reaching agreement about priorities and desired outcomes, there must be continuing efforts to share the existing knowledge and experience between agencies and disciplines.

We need to continue building up our picture of what services for this group of children and young people will look like. The starting-point must be the experiences of individual children and their families. Consultation with children and young people and their families will be important, but information from the individual assessments by professionals from all the relevant disciplines must also be drawn together.

One of the major obstacles to informed commissioning of services for children with learning disabilities and severe challenging behaviour has been the lack of adequate information. However, the requirement to produce Children's Services Plans DfEE(1996) should help to improve the situation since these plans will be strategic in nature and thus congruent in approach to NHS commissioning. Implementation of the SEN Code of Practice (DFE and Welsh Office, 1994) should also provide more comprehensive information than has been available up to now solely from the statementing process.

The assessment of local needs is the basis for commissioning. The process of 'needs assessment' has now been operating in the health services for the last four or five years and has three separate elements (NHSME, 1991):

▶ epidemiological information about the local population and prevalence of the conditions for which the services are being planned;

- national and local policy and professional opinion about service needs, together with the views of service users and carers;
- evidence, based on research, about the effectiveness of different treatments and types of service provision.

There is still some way to go before needs assessment fully incorporates all these elements in practice, particularly in relation to children with learning disabilities and severe challenging behaviour whose needs are so complex. However, the suggestion (Sutton, 1995) that local authorities should adopt the same needs assessment approach when drawing up their Children's Services Plans, should provide further impetus for comprehensive needs-based development of services.

8.7 Issues in contracting

Contracts for services for children with learning disabilities and challenging behaviour need to reflect the complexity, sensitivity and individual nature of the clinical and educational practice required for this work and the chronic nature of the disorders involved.

The current contracting system derives income from hospital admissions and new outpatient referrals. It gives little or no recognition to the need for out-patient follow-up and outreach services and this can actively undermine good paediatric and child-care practice. Contracting needs to develop greater flexibility which takes account of the following factors:

- Children will usually need detailed, long-term follow-up and decisions about workloads must reflect this.
- Follow-up may require more time than the initial consultation and may also involve a number of professionals such as social workers, psychologists, dieticians and the child's teacher.
- Close monitoring for secondary problems will be required as well as the provision of treatment and support in various settings such as the child's home and community.
- In some instances, a key worker or advocate for the child and/or the family may be needed.
- A flexible relationship between local services and the more highly specialised services is necessary so that each supports the other, according to the child's needs, over time.
- Attention to the needs of other family members may support them in caring for the child with severe challenging behaviour.

8.8 From extra-contractural referrals (ECRs) ... to a strategic approach

Although health authorities are being encouraged to move away from ECRs for individuals or small numbers of cases, there are circumstances which require commissioners to purchase very specialised services which operate on a supra-district, regional or even national basis.

ECRs pose problems for both commissioners and providers. Because placements are often one-offs, commissioners can find it difficult to influence the quality of provision for an individual and providers can end up having to operate contractual relationships with a (large) number of different purchasers. These concerns are likely to increase with the establishment of the new unitary authorities which because of their size are unlikely to have sufficient local demand for a specialist service.

This strengthens the case for developing a strategic approach, with commissioners and providers from different agencies working collaboratively.

Both purchasers and providers can benefit from a commissioned approach as set out in Williams and Richardson (1995).

Purchaser benefits include:

- greater input to quality control;
- more influence on continuity of care;
- access to information needed for future planning;
- greater influence on costs;
- can influence providers to disseminate skills through training and research.

Provider benefits include:

- enhanced financial security;
- greater ability to undertake financial and service planning for the future;
- more support for investment in training and research.

The advantages inherent in developing consistent commissioning approaches are obvious. Without this, services for the small numbers of children and young people with learning disabilities and severe challenging behaviour will remain in a precarious state in the internal market of our health and welfare system.

The foundation stone of commissioning is the assessment of the needs of these children by all agencies, together with evaluation of purchasing decisions and of the quality of the services purchased. The process of assessing needs – with expert input from relevant professionals and from the young people and their families – is a prerequisite for setting priorities and for ethical purchasing and commissioning decisions about services for children with learning disabilities and challenging behaviour, just as it is for the population as a whole (Klein, 1983).

8.9 Collaborative commissioning

Although, as noted above, health and local authorities have developed their commissioning/purchasing rôles along somewhat different lines, they are being actively encouraged to develop collaborative commissioning arrangements. This approach will be helped by the government decision making it mandatory for local authorities to produce Children's Services Plans in liaison with child health and education and will strengthen local authorities' strategic planning rôle along lines that are more congruent with those of the health service.

In the joint commissioning of specialised services it will be crucial to establish funding mechanisms. Handling of placements in specialised services will have to afford minimum disruption to the individuals receiving the service. Mechanisms for achieving this may include jointly funding a local service or agreeing a standard percentage split of costs for placements outside the district of residence.

Following a recent review of a commissioned service with a national catchment, the HAS/NHS Health Advisory Service (Williams and Richardson 1995) presented three possible models for health service commissioning. These are to establish:

- a number of district health authority consortia, each of which would contract for a proportion of the service;
- an underwriting mechanism administered by one or more DHA consortia or the NHS Executive itself. This would guarantee a level of income for each service, calculated on the basis of fixed and semi-fixed costs. Should the underwriting procedure be triggered in two consecutive years, a review of need would be undertaken to assess the requirement for the level of service offered;
- a lead commissioning authority for each such service that would contract on behalf of the whole country or a group of commissioners. The authority would be responsible for setting up and implementing an appropriate commissioning strategy. This would be based on assessment of need and involve quality assurance, monitoring of contract and outcomes and performance management.

Establishing any of these models requires constructive dialogue between commissioners and there may be a facilitative rôle for NHS Executive regional offices in this process.

Experience of collaborative commissioning models to date suggests a number of success criteria:

- a high level of trust in partner authorities;
- transparency in the contracting process; ie, concrete, unambiguous specification of service requirements attached to costs;
- good information on service use and costs;
- adopting a medium to long-term view on value for money;
- basing decisions on a robust needs assessment exercise.

Assessment and planning in social services

8.10 A common framework

Much of the evidence to the Committee referred to the Children Act 1989 and related guidance, reflecting the fact that this landmark legislation introduced the important principle of a common framework for services for all children. Many submissions pointed to the aspiration of services to meet the overarching requirement within the Children Act 1989 to safeguard and promote the welfare of the child and the corresponding duty to provide a range of services within the community for 'children in need'. For children with severe learning disabilities, one of the most significant aspects of the Act was their inclusion with other children; as children with severe disabilities but also 'children first'. Although many parents often felt overwhelmed by the stresses and difficulties they faced in everyday life, they made it clear to the Committee that they also wanted their children to be seen as 'children first'.

'My child is seen as a problem too difficult and too expensive. But she isn't a syndrome, she isn't a burden, she is my child. If you see her as a child, then it's easier to think of the services we need to stay together.' (A parent)

The Act incorporates a range of provisions to protect and support children in need (and their families) in a variety of settings, including family placements, day care, child minders and private, voluntary and local authority children's homes. This duty to care extends to children in hospitals, LEA residential establishments, independent and non-maintained schools, nursing homes and of course the family home.

The Children Act (1989) has led to increased expectations about support services, but a number of parents and professionals expressed their concerns to the Committee about the capacity of local authority services to meet the needs of children with complex and 'low incidence' disabilities. Some of the comments received by the Committee underline these hopes, fears and expectations.

'The Children Act (1989) made a real difference. We [as an authority] are now beginning to develop integrated assessment arrangements and to involve parents and disabled children in planning as well as in individual decision making. The Children Act (1989) challenged us all, not least because of competition for resources between statutory child protection procedures and wider support for children 'in need'.' (Social worker, child development centre)

'In some ways the Children Act (1989) has actually hindered the development of provision for children with learning disabilities and challenging behaviour. Social services departments have reorganised and changed their internal systems. Those staff with specific expertise have tended to move over to adult services. The Children Act (1989) initially oversimplified local authority responses to children with complex disabilities. Both the Act and the Guidance place too much emphasis upon desirability rather than on specific responsibilities.' (Parent representative, voluntary organisation)

'The implementation of the Children Act (1989) made very little difference to our Social services department's lack of policy – not only for children with challenging behaviour but for most services.' (Consultant psychiatrist)

'There is no reward for coping – but that is what the Children Act (1989) is all about – helping families to cope. If things don't get better, we'll be looking for a residential placement. At least that would keep us together.' (Parent)

8.11 A changing environment in children's services: purchaser/provider issues in planning

A universal theme running through evidence received by the Committee was that of assessment and planning arrangements and the extent to which these local arrangements took account of the needs of children with complex difficulties and provided clear messages for purchasers and planners about both current purchasing strategies and future planning procedures.

When the Committee was taking evidence, the government was consulting on the need for Children's Services Plans, to ensure that assessment and planning arrangements developed in the spirit of the Children Act (1989). This gave further encouragement to inter-agency collaboration. Children's Services Plans already existed informally in many local authorities but have assumed increasing importance in terms of partnership arrangements between health and local authorities. The guidance to accompany the now mandatory plans (DfEE/DoH, 1996) expects local authorities, as the lead agencies, to work with health authorities, NHS trusts, LEAs and governing bodies of grant maintained schools, voluntary organisations, the police and the probation service. Local authorities now need to demonstrate their strategic approach to providing children's services' (DfEE/DoH, 1996) based on:

- a reliable and comprehensive data-base;
- a thorough analysis of need and supply;
- the views of service users and the local community;
- consultation with other agencies;
- monitoring and feedback.

The process assumes the setting of standards and access to full and accurate information about services and performance. The guidance underlines the importance of local agencies developing shared definitions of need, reliable and accessible databases, agreed priorities and allocation of resources.

Although the purchasing of children's services is established practice in social services departments, formal contracting is a more recent development. An important strategic difference between children's and adult services is that local authorities cannot 'contract out' of their primary duties under Part III of the Children Act (1989) (services for children in need), unless they obtain specific statutory authority. But they are increasingly the enablers of service provision rather than the actual providers. This shift in rôle has produced its own challenges, not least the recognition that it is as important for local authorities to plan purchasing as it is for them to plan providing. The publication of Children's Services Plans should therefore enable local authorities to clarify the core services which they will provide and to define what they should purchase elsewhere. As few local authorities have their own services for children with challenging behaviour, the planning issue becomes of paramount importance – not only in the creation of positive working alliances with health and education, but also with other local authorities, in the specification and allocation of resources.

The Committee considers the Children's Services Planning framework to be particularly important as a context for planning specialist services for children with the most complex needs because it puts services for all children within a common framework. As Mansell noted, in the context of planning services for adults with challenging behaviour (1993), the reorientation away from health to social services has been positive in producing new patterns of community provision. But it has sometimes been simplistically interpreted as indicating that the health service has no rôle to play in the management of challenging behaviour. As a result, some small community services have therefore lacked the necessary expertise and support from the health service to support their users.

8.12 Mapping needs and resources

In a review of Children's Services Plans, Sutton (1995) for the National Children's Bureau and the DoH, notes that crossing boundaries in the assessment and mapping of need is a complex exercise. Needs can only be assessed jointly if agencies can agree a common definition of need. Sutton concluded that the most effective multi-agency approaches adopted in the first Children's Services Plans had:

- agreed definitions of need which were understandable across agency boundaries and which acknowledged the wide variations in levels and types of need among some groups of children;
- agreed measures of need and integrated assessment arrangements to facilitate both individual and collective planning and purchasing arrangements;
- reliable databases which were regularly updated;
- information about unit costs;

- prioritised short, medium and longer term planning objectives in conjunction with local users;
- had created mechanisms for joint commissioning, planning and working with agreed criteria for referral to and purchase of specialist services.

Reviewing Children's Services Plans, both Sutton (1995) and the DoH (1995) saw these as strategies for future joint commissioning and working. Although there had been initial anxieties that the Plans might be too general to permit constructive planning for children with low incidence disabilities, early analysis of the Plans showed that some authorities were aware of issues relating to challenging behaviour.

Several respondents to the Committee identified individual examples of planning which acknowledged the importance of specifying provision for children with significant behaviour difficulties:

- The creation of a multi-disciplinary team to work with local schools to identify children with emotional and behavioural difficulties, mental health problems and challenging behaviour at an early stage and to coordinate resources for a rapid response to avoid exclusions wherever possible.
- Local agreement between all three statutory services on 'risk factors' for emotional and behavioural difficulties or challenging behaviour and on the need to make earlier referrals for support. This Plan included specific arrangements for meeting the needs of the 200-300 children who at any one time might be regarded as being 'at serious risk'. The Plan set out agreed criteria for determining when to refer to a specialist service and for service level agreements with other authorities, where the child had a low-incidence disability which could not be met within the local or health authority's current purchasing arrangements.
- Better liaison with the relevant NHS trusts and child and adolescent mental health services through the local Children and Disability Teams.
- Service agreements with an adult services Behaviour Support Team, to provide professional advice to a children with disabilities team on the assessment of and provision for children with learning disabilities and severe challenging behaviour.

8.13 Assessment issues

'As a local authority, we are often overwhelmed by the multiplicity of assessment arrangements for some children. Assessment can be pro-active (ie looking for opportunities for services to respond more appropriately) or it can be reactive (endeavouring to ameliorate a current crisis). Increasingly social services departments are exhorted to think 'prevention' but we suffer from an unwillingness in many family services to actually specify 'challenging' or 'emotional and behavioural' difficulties. Reluctance to properly describe a child means that intervention is often late or inappropriate. Most importantly, we need to boost our own surveillance and screening arrangements and to keep records which enable us to truly 'track' children's progress. I am conscious that too many children end up in residential provision outside the authority because of reluctance to identify appropriately and to utilise specialist services. The concept of 'social' or 'medical' models of care can be unhelpful when early referral to an appropriate specialist unit in the health service might have avoided a residential placement.' (Manager, children with disabilities team)

'As a parent, we came to dread assessment. It felt as if it was used to screen us out of services, not to welcome us in. Most importantly we often felt that referral to another service (particularly between health and social services) was seen as a failure for all of us and our child. We could not understand why community nurses with learning disability experience seem no longer to work with children – what we all needed (social services too) was some hands-on practical help. Finally we got to a specialist unit – providing a regional if not a national service. They were able to really help, not just in understanding our child but in supporting our local services to do so as well. Challenging behaviour like our son has is really such a rarity – why are 'specialists' so unpopular in some services? If I had cancer, I would know that the best help for me and my local carers would probably come from a specialist hospital. It is not institutionalisation we are talking about any more, it's supporting the community.' (Parent of a twelve year old autistic son)

Many respondents to the Committee emphasised the often inadequate integration of assessments within local planning and purchasing protocols for children with challenging behaviour. A further significant particular problem was the multiplicity of assessment arrangements which might be used sometimes simultaneously. The DoH guidance on child protection (1993) and on child and adolescent health(1995) identify a range of different assessments for children with disabilities, special educational needs, health, or mental health problems, including:

▶ developmental/health assessment
▶ psychometric assessment
▶ special educational needs assessment
▶ parenting assessment
▶ family assessment
▶ risk assessment
▶ access (for a specific service) assessment

Some of these assessment approaches focus primarily on the competencies of the family, some focus specifically on aspects of a child's overall health and development and some will form part of screening and surveillance arrangements which apply to all children. Others address the child's specific needs. In most instances there will be a 'lead' agency but there is a corresponding need for inter-agency collaboration and much fragmentation in reality.

Several respondents referred to the Audit Commission's report (1994) on cooperation between health and social services for children 'in need'. The Commission noted the importance of matching levels of assessment to levels of need and envisaged Children's Services Plans as providing a local framework for greater specificity about assessment; allocation of resources to meet identified need; and more focused and appropriate use of specialist services for children with significant behavioural or other special needs. To achieve such an outcome, the Commission recommended a 'tiered' approach to services in order to rationalise assessment arrangements and ensure prompt referrals to specialist services when required.

The DoH,(1995) also adopts a 'tiered' approach to assessment and need which reflects the management approach advocated by a number of the Committee's respondents. This suggests that:

Tier one provides a primary level service: for example, teachers, GPs, health visitors community nurses and social services.

Tier two provides services through specific professionals who will usually be linked to other services (though not necessarily as part of a specialist team). These might include clinical psychologists, community paediatricians, educational psychologists. Their rôle will include training and consultation for other professionals (particularly those in Tier l); assessment and some outreach services to those working in the community.

Tier three offers specialist services for those with more severe disabilities or complex special needs. The tier will generally offer a multi-disciplinary team or service, usually with a specialist remit and providing a range of assessment, intervention and referral services.

Tier four will meet the needs of children with the most challenging or difficult behaviour and will access children to infrequently used and very specialist services. At this level, the services will be provided on a supra-district level and could involve a residential placement. Services are likely to involve joint commissioning and possible service-level agreements with neighbouring authorities or NHS trusts.

Most children with learning disabilities will be seen and supported at Tiers One and Two. But when the child has challenging behaviour or more complex needs, he or she may be referred to Tier Three or Four.

Assessment of children with learning disabilities and severe challenging behaviour will include the existing assessment arrangements which would apply to any child with special needs (ie statutory assessment under the Education Act, 1996) and will also need to take account of the wide range of factors which may affect the health or behaviour of the child such as:

▶ family disadvantage;
▶ poor parenting skills;

- chronic physical illness;
- learning difficulties, language or communication problems;
- physical, sexual or emotional abuse;
- experience of sudden transition
- specific syndromes.

This Committee, like the Mansell Committee before them, acknowledge that the purpose of assessment of challenging behaviour needs to be clarified. Challenging behaviour will occur because of a complex mix of environmental and individual circumstances. Hence appropriate referrals to and utilisation of specialist services will be ineffective without a recognition that the maintenance of any intervention will necessitate improving the quality and responsiveness of mainstream services for children with disabilities. A number of respondents referred to Mansell (1993) and the underlying message that crisis intervention was only a temporary solution. As Mansell notes (1993: 25):

'If they [services in the community for people with learning disabilities] develop the capacity to work with people who present challenges in small local services, they will keep the size of the problem to a minimum and they will provide a good service to individuals in both their mainstream and specialised services. If local services are not developed, then a trickle of expensive out-of-area placements will become a rush as more people are excluded from mainstream community services by being defined as unmanageable. More money will be tied up in less good services.'

During its work, the Committee was aware of increasing evidence of children with severe challenging behaviour and learning disabilities being placed in out-of-area residential placements. Whilst in some instances this reflected a positive choice for a very challenging child, in other circumstances it reflected a slow process of attrition, in which the child had been increasingly excluded from local services and the family had broken down. In most cases of which we were aware, these emergency placements reflected crisis judgements rather than coherent assessment and planning. In many instances, parents told us that they had no alternative but to ask for a residential placement, because no community resources existed. Some members of the Council for Disabled Children (Russell 1995) asked to comment on Children's Services Plans and challenging behaviour, endorsed Mansell, noting that:

'A key indicator for success at local level should be integrated assessment arrangements, with individual care plans and specified targets for regular review. Secondly, any plan (whether the new Children's Services Plans or Community Care Plans) should have to state:

- How many children were placed in 'out of area' schools or other provision during the year?
- What was the purpose of their placement and how will it be monitored?
- How many placements reflected local arrangements breaking down, pressures on families and 'crisis' action?
- What is the cost of 'away' placements? And what would the equivalent service have cost if provided in the community?
- How does the local authority distinguish between 'emotional and behavioural difficulties'; 'challenging behaviour' and 'mental health problems'? Should there be an authority-wide strategy for behaviour issues, however defined?
- How can we ensure that families and carers (and mainstream professionals and carers) get the support they need? A child's behaviour can affect a whole family. Who is the user and do we respect families who just about cope?
- As organisations concerned with children and families, we are also concerned about the children who should challenge us – the withdrawn, the isolated, the unhappy children. Some families feel that the tariff for a service is too often only attached to the troublesome and not to the troubled children.'

Many parents, like local and health authorities, were concerned about the question of 'value for money'. A community paediatrician working in a child development centre with 'early identification' programmes for children with a range of behavioural difficulties, commented that:

> 'Value for money is so often seen in terms of short-term solutions to long-term problems. We consider that an 'eco-behavioural' approach makes the most sense. That is to say, you must see the child in the context of his or her immediate environment, the local community and of course his or her individual special needs. When working with very young children, we are aware that much of the research gives equivocal messages about the optimum model for early intervention. But we do know from research and our own practice that helping the families of young children with special needs helps the children. This is why individual assessment must be linked to team approaches. In working as a team, we also have to acknowledge that some young children are very challenging indeed and simple containment becomes increasingly unrealistic. We must regard the growing numbers of exclusions as a warning sign of the need to take challenging behaviour seriously right from the start, when intervention may be practicable. We must also develop effective 'risk indicators' to enable us to target scarce resources more effectively.'

Several submissions to the Committee highlighted the importance of developing locally agreed:

- 'risk factors' for the early identification of potentially challenging behaviour in young children;
- assessment arrangements for children with learning disabilities and severe challenging behaviour;
- criteria for referral of children to specialist (usually out of area) services for further assessment or treatment;
- protocols for the joint funding/joint commissioning of certain specialist services which cannot be provided on a local basis, with monitoring and review arrangements specified throughout all three statutory agencies;
- policies for family support services which acknowledge that some children may be very challenging and that respite and other provision may need to be expanded and supported to meet these children's additional needs.

One local authority team for children with disabilities emphasised the 'cultural revolution' for many social services departments in expanding the capacity of their child and family services to meet the needs of children with challenging behaviour. This team had determined that it must 'learn from its own experience' and was tracking six children with challenging behaviour and learning disabilities over the coming year in order to identify positive (and negative) factors in local services.

8.14 Building consumers into the planning framework

Children's Services Plans (as with Community Care plans) theoretically build consumer consultation into the planning process. We were made aware of a number of local authority planning forums which involved parents and carers. Some were exploring ways of involving children and young people. But many identified the difficulties of actually involving parents of children with learning disabilities and associated challenging behaviour in this process. One manager from a local authority team for children with disabilities noted that although parent involvement was a priority, there had been problems authorising this.

> 'We have a parents' forum and this has a considerable influence on our planning processes. At the moment, we are looking at streamlining assessment arrangements so that we only need to consider what we actually need to know. This is challenging to all concerned, but the parents now understand our dilemma – we hesitate between 'positive images of disability' and 'needing to allocate resources appropriately and equitably'. Somewhere between the two is a workable and acceptable arrangement. But we are conscious that in this process we have a minority, sometimes no, parents of children with challenging behaviour. They are often too tired, too busy – or sometimes too depressed – to join us. So we are now holding regular consultative meetings with them. This has had a very positive impact on our commissioners of services. If they do not know what parents want, they can neither commission – nor fully review – what they are offering. We hope that our 'value' for money marker two years from now will be that we have reinvested more in community provision and our 'out-of-county' purchases will reflect real and specialist need.'

Another social services respondent commented that he was using the development of a register of children with disabilities as an opportunity to get parents of children with low-incidence disabilities into the planning system. He had identified ten children with learning disabilities and associated significant behaviour difficulties (noting that although very similar, only four were actually described as having challenging behaviour). He was working with these families individually as they found it difficult to attend meetings to ensure that their wishes and feelings were built into the planning system. He observed that 'isolation, fragmentation and chance' seemed to characterise their access to services:

'A particular problem with some parents was that they were referred to specialist services and received very good advice and treatment. But when the child returned home, they were isolated. Sometimes schools and family support services refused to accept the child on the basis of his or her former reputation. The families wished to have (and now will receive) 'back-up' support in the community. Schools, nurseries and other providers know they have access to 'fast-track' advice and there is more confidence in the system.'

The authority was now planning a behaviour support team to provide specialist input into a wide range of services.

This very specific consultation with parents underlined the importance of building consumer views into planning and the dangers of investing in specialist services without parallel investment in the community services to which the child would return.

Recommendations

Core Recommendations

▶ Purchasing and commissioning plans should be developed from the principle that children with learning disabilities and severe challenging behaviour are 'children first' and should have access to positive experiences and care within their local communities wherever possible.

▶ The highly specialised components of services for these children should be commissioned as part of a continuum of provision that takes account not only of their special needs but also of their overall needs as children and the likelihood of their continuing long-term needs during childhood, through the transition and into adulthood.

Collaboration

▶ Commissioners, purchasers and providers should develop service specifications for children with learning disabilities and severe challenging behaviour which are based on shared understanding and definitions of need in order to develop more integrated provision.

▶ The needs of children with learning disabilities and severe challenging behaviour should be included in a commissioning framework jointly developed and agreed by the health, social services and education authorities.

▶ Joint purchasing and commissioning arrangements that ensure that children have access to a range of specialist provision which is otherwise unlikely to be viable within a single locality should be developed.

▶ Flexible purchasing and contracting arrangements should to be developed which allow for consultation and liaison work by specialist staff with a child's local and primary caregivers, so as to support and encourage their competence and confidence and reduce the likelihood of long-term residential placement.

Specialist services

▶ Purchasers and commissioners should recognise that many of these children will require highly expert and specialist support to sustain them and their families within the local community.

▶ Purchasing and contracting arrangements should ensure the continuing viability of the specialist resources that may be needed by these children and their families, which should include funding for the evaluation and development of specialist services.

▶ Purchasing arrangements should indicate services for children with learning disabilities and severe challenging behaviour with services for other groups of children who may require highly specialised approaches.

References

Audit Commission (1994) Seen but not Heard: Co-ordinating Community Child Health and Social Services for Children in Need. Audit Commission.

Verrier Jones K and Lissauer J J (1995) Tertiary Services for Children and Young People: A Guide for purchase Provision and Planning of Specialist Services for Sick Children. The Royal College of Paediatrics and Child Health.

Council for Disabled Children (1996) Commenting on children's plans a disability perspective. Unpublished discussion paper available from the Council for Disabled Children.

Department of Health (1991) Working Together under the Children Act 1989. HMSO.

Department of Health/Department for Education and Employment (1996) Children's Service Planning Guidance. DoH/DfEE.

DoH (1995) A Handbook on Child and Adolescent Mental Health. Health of the Nation/DoH.

Klein R (1993) Rationality and rationing diffused or concentrated decision making. In Rationing of Health Care in Medicine. Ed. M Tunbridge. Royal College of Physicians.

Kurtz Z, Thornes R and Volkind S (1994) Services for the Mental Health of Children and Young People in England A National Survey. Department of Health/South Thames Regional Health Authority.

NHS Management Executive (1991) Assessing Health Care Needs: A DHA Project Discussion Paper. Department of Health.

NHSME (1993) Contracting for Specialist Services: A Practical Guide. NHSME.

Social Services Inspectorate (SS1) (1995) Children's Services Plans: An analysis of Children's Services Plans 1993/4. Social Services Inspectorate.

Sutton P (1995) Crossing the Boundaries: A Discussion of Children's Services Plans. National Children's Bureau.

Williams R and Richardson G (eds) (1995) Together We Stand: The Commissing Role and Management of Child and Adolescent Mental Health Services. Health Advisory Service/HMSO.

Epilogue

The past decade has seen major changes in children's services. The implementation of the Children Act 1989 and the Education Act 1993 created a new optimism and a spirit of entitlement to good quality services for all children with disabilities amongst parents, purchasers and providers alike. In the same period we have seen an ongoing debate about inclusion and participation for all children in our communities. There has been a welcome focus upon 'partnership with parents' and a refocusing of local authority services away from crisis intervention towards family support and preventive strategies. But there has also been a corresponding (and often negative) debate about difficult and disruptive children in schools and a less tolerant attitude generally to children or families who appear in any way 'different'.

Children with learning disabilities and severe challenging behaviour are probably amongst the most vulnerable children in our society. They may not fit easily into existing systems or services and their complex needs may not be acknowledged. As one parent commented to us during the course of our discussions,

'Our children are often seen as just too expensive. Or rather they are seen as expensive without giving 'value for money'. But they do repay investment very well! My son has received excellent help, his school, we as parents have all had advice and support and we have felt confident that we were doing a good job. It hasn't been easy, but it's been worth it. Paul is our son, we love him and we wanted him to have an ordinary life. Not much to ask for, an ordinary life – but it can seem as distant as the moon when you are struggling to live with challenging behaviour. Let's publicly value our good services – it's too easy to forget challenging behaviour and we parents are often too tired to act as advocates.'

Paul's mother reminds us that children with challenging behaviour are family members and the Committee was made very aware that these children are loved and valued; that they can make progress and that there are some innovative and effective services. However, we were also aware that in many respects children with learning disabilities and severe challenging behaviour and their families form a silent minority. Some families felt that they desperately needed services like short-term care the most, but were ironically least likely to get it because of their child's behaviour. Many families felt that services were fragmented, difficult to access and often unsuitable for their needs.

A key issue within the work of this Committee and that of the Department of Health's (DoH) review of services for adults with learning disabilities and challenging behaviour (The Mansell Report, 1993) was that of strategic planning. The welcome shift towards 'ordinary life' and local services has not always benefited children and adults with learning disabilities with the most challenging needs. Children with learning disabilities and challenging behaviour can be expensive. But, as the Audit Commission commented (1994), in its report Seen but not Heard (a review of local authority services for children 'in need'):

'Two billion pounds per annum is spent on children's services, but little is known about the impact – services should focus on needs and their impact should be evaluated.'

As ever in human services, there are threats and opportunities. Like this Committee, the Audit Commission noted that children with the greatest need frequently received the most poorly coordinated services, without significant evidence of effective assessment and strategic planning and with many dissatisfied parents. However, during our work, we were aware of a significant shift in policy development towards strategic planning and a recognition that all children should receive services within a common policy framework.

The implementation of Children's Services Plans in 1996 gave a long-awaited impetus to integrated local and health authority planning. The NHS Executive prioritised 'children in need' within its purchasing guidance for children's services. OFSTED (1996) saw evidence of positive impact from implementation of the Code of Practice, in terms of schools and LEAs working closely and more coherently together in the identification of and provision for children with special educational needs.

In 1997 we are likely to see a new Education Bill, which will require LEAs for the first time to have clearly articulated behaviour policies. Although these policies will be primarily directed at the 'pupils with problems' whose exclusion from school has preoccupied the media for many months, they also offer opportunities to ensure that challenging behaviour is reconceptualised as everybody's responsibility.

As a Committee, we were impressed by the achievements of many families and those working with them. We were aware of the tremendous task of ensuring that this group of children were, indeed, seen as 'children first', whilst having access to a full range of specialist services as appropriate. We are also aware that, as the Mental Health Foundation (1996) noted in its report, Building Expectations: Opportunities for Services for People with a Learning Disability:

'The next generation of parents and children will not be the same as those of today. There will be no safety net of long-stay hospitals and children will be more a part of their local communities. People with learning disabilities will be affected by the wider disability movement and its emphasis on choices, rights and participation.' (section 9.62)

Meeting the needs of this next generation of children and parents will be challenging. As noted above, we see the growing commitment to a strategic and integrated approach to assessment and commissioning as critical in order to avoid fragmentation, duplication and isolation. The issue of resources will not go away, but – as this report highlights – resources could and should be targeted more effectively. Targeting will not be possible without a clear policy framework and within our report we are aware of a number of key issues to be addressed in developing greater quality, clarity and cohesion in service responses to children with learning disabilities and challenging behaviour:

▶ First, we still know very little about the feasibility of earlier identification and intervention for children with severe challenging behaviour. There are important issues about investment in research and evaluation and in developing and disseminating interesting and innovative approaches to working with children with learning disabilities and severe challenging behaviour.

▶ Secondly, many families complained to us of 'feast or famine' in terms of locally available services and support. We cannot sufficiently underline the importance of envisaging severe challenging behaviour as everyone's business and ensuring that the needs of this group of children are fully addressed within Children's Services Planning arrangements and the purchasing and commissioning priorities of the relevant Health Authority.

▶ Thirdly, the general commitment to local community-based services is unlikely to be effective for children with learning disabilities and challenging behaviour unless central government policy provides assistance in informing and encouraging a national debate about how best to develop:

local policy and practice for children with severe challenging behaviour within the context of wider developments for children 'in need' within the area; and

an appropriate balance between inclusive and specialist services for children with the most complex needs;

investment in training and professional development to ensure sufficient availability of specialist staff and greater competence and confidence within staff working in community services.

▶ Fourthly, we must not forget the parents and children and ensure that their wishes, feelings and perceptions of services are firmly built into local planning and purchasing arrangements. Many families of children with severe challenging behaviour see themselves as a 'forgotten minority', too tired and often too isolated to contribute to the wider network of parent organisations. We need to be creative in ascertaining their views, in seeing them as real partners in their child's care and development and acknowledging the real practical and emotional impact of living with severe challenging behaviour on a day-to-day basis.

▶ Finally and by no means least, we should acknowledge the importance of investment in 'the next generation'. As the Mansell Report noted, we must understand children with learning disabilities and severe challenging behaviour, if we are to respond appropriately to adults. In children's services we have the additional resource of the education system and the real possibility of developing new approaches to the identification and assessment of severe challenging behaviour which balance:

access to services which are designed to promote the 'well being' of all children with:

access to appropriate specialist services, including services provided on an out-reach basis to community services.

The transition to a valued adult life is probably one of the greatest transitions that any of us make. It necessitates changes in family relationships; the development of a new adult rôle; important discussions about employment opportunities and adult relationships and the recognition with greater personal autonomy of responsibilities as well as rights. Children with learning disabilities and severe challenging behaviour also make these transitions, but the extent to which they achieve the 'markers' of adult life will be very variable. The Committee heard from some families and from professional services about the challenge of the current requirement to provide a 'transition plan' at the fourteen-plus statutory annual review as required by the Code of Practice and the 1996 Education Act. As one parent put it:

'My son will become an adult, whether we like it or not. But he is unlikely to be able to achieve the 'ordinary life' which is the primary aspiration of so many local authority community care plans. His life options may well diminish, because we will lose our familiar and trusted child health services; our essential local authority respite care; the day-to-day commitment and shared learning of David's school.

We may grumble about children's services, about the lack of resources, the endless assessments – but we know where we are! Where will David and I be when he leaves school? He has had a childhood, he has stayed in his local community. But not for long. I don't want to be one of the faceless statistics fighting their local authority for a residential placement. I don't want to go to judicial review for a service. I want an honest and open debate about challenging behaviour as a continuing factor in all our lives. Let's face it, we are investing in all our futures. Please don't forget us!'

We hope that this report will contribute to an important debate and that it will create greater awareness about the minority of children with learning disabilities and severe challenging behaviour who are living in our local communities. These children are sometimes invisible within local planning arrangements. But their visibility will be marked and the challenges considerable if we do not adopt a life-cycle approach to the early identification, assessment and management of severe challenging behaviour, invest in families and services and ensure that these children (and adults) are clearly identified within all local planning structures.

Overarching recommendations

▶ Children with learning disabilities and severe challenging behaviour should have access to a range of services, including specialist provision, to help them lead positive and valued lives within their families and local communities and enjoy the range of education, play and leisure opportunities available to other children.

▶ Policies, plans and services for children with learning disabilities and severe challenging behaviour and their families should reflect the cultural, racial and religious diversity of society, take account of the differing patterns of family life and acknowledge the individual experiences and aspirations of children and their families.

▶ Local commissioning and purchasing plans, including Children's Services Plans, should include specific reference to the needs of children with learning disabilities and severe challenging behaviour and should set out clear local arrangements for inter-agency collaboration.

▶ All multi-agency work, including purchasing and commissioning of services, should be based on shared and agreed definitions of 'severe challenging behaviour'.

▶ Children with learning disabilities and severe challenging behaviour should have access to a comprehensive, multi-disciplinary and properly co-ordinated assessment of their individual needs, regardless of which service has been approached initially.

▶ Children with learning disabilities and severe challenging behaviour should have access to services which are child-centred, take account of their individual needs and are in the child's best interests.

▶ Purchasers and providers should recognise that children with severe challenging behaviour will often require specialist services on a continuing and long-term basis and allocation of resources should take this into account.

▶ All interventions should be based on partnership between families and service providers and on an interpretation of the law which is sensitive to the demands and needs of those families, whilst at the same time promoting what is the paramount interest of the children. Interventions should seek to enhance the competence and confidence of families and carers in supporting children with severe challenging behaviour.

▶ The DoH and DfEE should jointly establish nationally agreed and enforceable minimum standards for the training and qualifications of staff working in health, social care, education and other services for children with severe challenging behaviour.

▶ Wherever possible, children should be enabled to remain at home, using local facilities, but if a residential placement is considered necessary, commissioners should actively seek appropriate provision which is as local as possible.

▶ Government and other funding bodies should invest in research to inform the development of quality services for children with severe challenging behaviour and to ensure that scarce resources are used effectively.

▶ Government departments should collaborate to ensure that policy and guidance with reference to children with challenging behaviour issued by individual departments provides a coherent and consistent framework for local service planning and development.

APPENDIX 1: The conduct and activities of the Committee

The Committee was convened in October 1993 to investigate current patterns of provision for children and young people with learning disabilities and severe challenging behaviour and to make recommendations for action. The definitions used by the Committee are set out in chapter 2.

The Committee met regularly over a period of three and a half years and took oral evidence from a range of expert witnesses at a consultation seminar. 1600 requests for written evidence were sent out to a wide range of organisations and individuals. Social services and education departments, health authorities, trusts, professional organisations and the voluntary sector were approached. Parents and siblings also responded to questionnaires and the Committee was able to seek their views through parent meetings, schools and other services working directly with families. Some of the evidence from families has been incorporated as quotations within the main text of the report because of the valuable insights and personal perspectives which it offers on the impact on family life of severe challenging behaviour.

The members of the Committee brought their own extensive knowledge and experience of services for children and young people with learning disabilities and severe challenging behaviour. Some members of the Committee made additional site visits to inform themselves about particular aspects of the care and education of these children and young people.

Because of the Committee's concern to identify preventive or early intervention strategies for young children with learning disabilities and severe challenging behaviour (and the lack of information in this area), Professor Chris Kiernan, director of the Hester Adrian Research Centre, was commissioned to carry out a literature search on early intervention to inform the Committee's work.

The Mental Health Foundation organised a conference in October 1995 to enable the Committee to share some early reflections on its work with an audience of professionals, managers and parents. This conference provided an important opportunity to clarify and to develop a number of themes in the subsequent report.

The different sections of the report were drafted by individual members of the Committee with particular expertise in that area, after a full and open discussion within the full Committee. The Committee also invited a number of critical readers to comment on the various drafts. The final report is edited by Alison Wertheimer.

APPENDIX 2

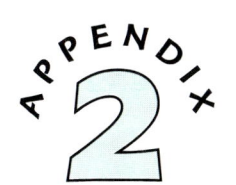

Individuals and organisations submitting evidence

Oral evidence

Dr Tom Berney	Consultant Psychiatrist, Prudhoe Hospital, Northumberland
Denise Weir	Head of Care, Radlett Lodge School
Richard Rollinson	Headteacher, The Mulberry Bush School, Witney, Oxon
Valerie Sinason	Consultant Psychiatrist, The Tavistock Centre, London
Peter Newell	Coordinator, EPOCH, London
Marion Cornick	Principal, Lodden School, Hants
Professor Rory Nicol	Professor of Child Psychiatry, University of Leicester
Dr Glynis Murphy	Senior Lecturer, Tizard Centre, University of Kent
Professor Eric Emerson	Professor of Clinical Psychology in Intellectual disability, Hester Adrian Research Centre, University of Manchester

Written evidence, individuals and organisations

May Anderson	Project Leader, Carraigfoyle Paediatric Support Team (Barnados), Northern Ireland
Dr M Bambrick	Consultant Psychiatrist, Southern Derbyshire Community Health Services Trust
Dr Jane Bernal	Senior Lecturer and Consultant Psychiatrist, St George's Hospital Medical School
Dr Tom Berney	Consultant Psychiatrist, Prudhoe Hospital
Dr Nick Bouras	UMDS Guy's & St Thomas's Hospital
BPA Working Party	(Services for Children and Adolescents with Learning Disabilities) Report
Linda Buchan	Consultant Psychologist, Child & Family Support Service
Hilary Cass	Harper House Children's Service
Karen J Castle	(Principal Development Officer, Children & Young People with Disabilities), Social Services Department, Cardiff, Children's Intensive Support Service
Linda Clough	Community Nurse, St Helens & Knowsley
Department of Health	Richmond House
Mrs Asha Desai	Head of Clinical Psychology, Community Team for People with Learning Disabilities, Hounslow
Janet Edmonds	Purchasing Assistant, Bromley Health Authority (& FHSA)
Annabelle Fenwick	Principal Clinical Psychologist
Rita Flanagan	Staff Development & Training Manager, Barnados Liverpool
Joyce Fletcher	Deputy Head, Pens Meadow School
Judy Fox	Clinical Psychologist, Avalon NHS Trust
Mr A Furze	Headteacher, Harborough School, London N19
Barry Hall	
Annette Hames	Clinical Psychologist, Community Team Learning Disability, Newcastle-upon-Tyne
Dr Josephine Hammond	St George's Healthcare
Tina Harvey	Headteacher, St Ann's School, Morden
Dr A Hauck	Consultant Psychiatrist, Leicester Firth Hospital
Professor Peter Hill	St George's Hospital Medical School
Dr Patricia Howlin	Consultant Psychologist, St George's Hospital Medical School
Deborah Hunt	Clinical Manager, Learning Disabilities Services, Hinchingbrooke Health Care

Dr Tom Hutchison	Consultant Community Paediatrician, Bath West NHS Trust
Professor Chris Kiernan	Director, Hester Adrian Research Centre
Chris Kippax	Dorset Social Services
Dr Zarrina Kurtz	Consultant in Public Health and Health Policy
Penny Lacey	University of Birmingham
Margaret Lally	Early Years Consultant
Dr Mary Lindsey	Cornwall & Isles of Scilly, Learning Disabilities NHS Trust
Chris Lock	Policy & Administration Director, MacIntyre Care
Carol MacDonald	Behavioural Support Team, East Berkshire NHS Trust
Dr B Male	Consultant Psychiatrist, Chichester Priority Service NHS Trust
Ruth Marchant	Chailey Heritage
Stuart Marpole	Service Development Officer (Children & Families), Norfolk County Council Social Services Department
B McGinnis	Special Adviser, MENCAP
Marian E McGowan	Consultant Community Paedrician, Merton & Sutton NHS Trust
Dr Ian McKinlay	Senior Lecturer in Community Child Health
Mr M Miles	
Richard Mills	Director of Services, National Autistic Society
J R Moore	Chair Advisory Speciality Committee on Paediatrics
Dean Morris	Children's Intensive Support Service
Professor Rory Nicol	Professor of Child Psychiatry, University of Leicester
Norfolk Social Services	
Norfolk Education Authority	
East Norfolk Health Commission	
Ovingdean Hall School	Brighton
Chris Roberts	Consultant Clinical Psychologist, Harrow Learning Disability Team
Carol Robinson	Senior Research Fellow, Norah Fry Research Centre
John Robinson	Directorate of Mental Health, Learning Disabilities, Hartlepool & South Easington Health Care
Philippa Russell	Director, Council for Disabled Children
Jean Score	Special Needs Coordinator Children, Lewisham Social Services
John Sharich	Consultant Clinical Psychologist, Oxfordshire Learning Disability NHS Trust
Dr E C Sheldrick	Consultant Psychiatrist, The Maudsley Hospital
Professor David Sines	Chair, Society of Nursing for People with a Learning Disability, Royal College of Nursing
Rosemary Singh	Chartered Clinical Psychologist, City & East London Family & Community Health Services
David Smith	Nurse Team Leader, The Maudsley Hospital
Jenny Summerfield	Planning & Development Officer, City of Coventry Social Services
Surrey Education Services	Surrey County Council
The University of York	Department of Social Policy & Social Work
Martin Van Tol	Commissioner for Children & Families, South Essex Health Authority
Alexander Toogood	Team Manager, Intensive Support Team, Clwyd
Dr Tyrone Trower	Lecturer in Child Psychiatry & Chair of Learning Disability Team, University of Leicester
Geoff Upton	Dorset Health Commission
Barbara Wallace	Health Promotion Strategist, South of Tyne Commission
Beck Williams	Senior Nurse/Behavioural Therapist, Gwynedd Community Health Trust
Andrea Wolf	Committees Officer, Royal College of Psychiatrists
Mrs F Wood	Villa Real School, Consett, Co. Durham